CANCER
PREVENTION AND NEW BREAKTHROUGH CURES

Virginia Becker

ISBN 1-58500-001-9

This book is printed on acid free paper.

1stBooks – Rev. 4/23/01

ABOUT THE BOOK

This is an expose of why there is so much cancer in our country. It also details preventive measures to reduce one's risk of getting cancer.

IN MEMORIAM

Hazel O'Donovan
Friend
Fellow Teacher
Nutritionist
Inspiration

Mary Jane Rohr-Hynes
Beloved Sister
Best Friend

TABLE OF CONTENTS

CHAPTER ONE

The Cancer Culture

We live, in the United States of America, in a cancer culture. Factors in our way of life have caused the rate of cancer to increase. America is losing the war on cancer.

The extent of this plague is easy to discern. It is assumed that we will get cancer. This is revealed in advice such as: "Early detection helps survival chances." Ads appear in magazines proclaiming "You can beat cancer– I'm living proof." Cancer has increased in children so there are cancer camps where dying children can have "fun." Obituary notices announce "Mary Smith, age 40, died after a long courageous battle with cancer."

What accounts for this tragic state of affairs? Why does our way of life promote such a devastating deadly disease? There has to be a logical explanation for the sad situation. Dr. E. Boyland, a cancer specialist, estimated:

"Not more than 5 percent of human cancer is due to viruses, less than 5 percent to

Radiation, and some 90 percent is due to chemicals. We do not know how much is due to endogenous carcinogens, how much is due to environmental factors." [1]

It is safe to assume that much human cancer is caused by carcinogens, cancer triggering agents, in food, water, drugs, cosmetics and in the air we breath. Chemicals saturate our food to such excess that Americans eat more chemicalized food than any people on earth. And Americans have more degenerative disease than any people on earth.

The average American eats one hundred and forty pounds of

1

chemical additives every year. Chemical companies sell billions of dollars worth of their lethal additives yearly to agribusiness. While the cancer plague stalks us, we are studied to death. When governments in other countries ban carcinogens, our Congress passed Acts requiring the Food and Drug Administration (hereinafter the FDA) to "study and label" them add to this irony– the fact that the studies are not released to the public. Information is withheld from the people whose tax dollars financed the studies.

In 1966 Sweden hosted an international conference on mercury. Five United States scientists were there. Mercury, which is odorless and tasteless, builds up in body tissues. It is deadly. There should be a zero limit for mercury in food. Since mercury can damage the nervous system, it is small wonder so many Americans are prescribed tranquilizers. Sweden banned mercury. America did not.

Our government agencies established to protect the health of consumers have failed to do so. They service agribusiness. What is agribusiness? How did it grow so fast? It is now the richest, most powerful industry in the United States of America. How did it grow with no restraint? Why is it still unrestrained?

Corporations that process, market, and produce farm commodities are agribusiness. Meat packers and seed companies are agribusiness. So are the chemical companies that sell food additives and pesticides. [2]

Agribusiness grew, unrestrained, at a furious pace because government agencies, which are supposed to be responsible for the regulation of such industries, are not enforcing the laws, which were enacted to regulate them. The two agencies responsible for monitoring agribusiness and enforcing consumer protection laws are the FDA and the United States Department of Agriculture (hereinafter referred to as USDA).

A clear example of the malfeasance and nonfeasance of administrators in these agencies is the filth allowed in meat today. The oldest Federal regulation agency for food was established in 1865 to regulate meat. However, the real power over meat production and marketing was in the meat conglomerates. Consumers realized this and fought for clean meat. They won a victory with the Wholesome Meat Act of 1967. It was an empty victory. It has never been enforced.

The food industry must be controlled by law. It has never regulated itself. It never will. Dr. Harvey Wiley said, "The American

2

people are being steadily poisoned by the dangerous chemicals being added to food with reckless abandon."[3] Because of his sacrifices and hard fought crusade, Congress passed the Food and Drug Act in 1906. On January 1, 1907 the FDA was founded to be responsible for safe food and drugs. It is a branch of health, education, and welfare (hereinafter to be known as H.E.W.).

The FDA is supposed to check the method of food manufacture, conduct hearings, set limits on additives and dirt, approve drug applications, seize and recall food, drugs, and cosmetics deemed unsafe and watchdog agribusiness. Its performance has been and still is a farce– a fraud. It has withheld information. It has deceived and betrayed the people.

For example, Dr. W.C. Hueper, Chief of the Environmental Cancer Section of the National Cancer Institute, wrote an article to alert people that chemicals in food can cause cancer. The FDA stopped publication of his article.[4] In the 1960's the FDA was busy raiding health food stores to confiscate vitamins. It should have been regulating agribusiness.

The tragic pollution of our food, water, and drugs with carcinogens is not the whole story of why we live in a cancer culture. The air we breathe is now polluted.

The New York City Department of Sanitation started a garbage dump and landfill in Pelham Bay Park in the 1960's. The site was to be used for household trash. Soon illegal industrial waste was dumped there. Waste oils, PCBs, cyanides and solvents were thrown into this landfill in 1978, filled to capacity, the dump was closed.

Meanwhile, in an adjacent neighborhood, twelve children were diagnosed with leukemia. When Kerri Nonnon was stricken, her mother Patricia Nonnon, investigated the dump. New York City issued a report that the dump was safe. New York State Department of Environmental Conservation labeled Pelham Bay a toxic waste danger spot, but did not schedule a clean up. 1.1 million gallons of waste had been dumped there. Now the statistics came in. There were 75 cancers, 12 leukemia cases, 6 cases of lupus, 6 cases of autism, 7 rare blood disease cases, 47 cases of multiple sclerosis. NUT UNTIL 1990 DID THE CLEAN UP START.

While we are losing the war on cancer, how has the American Medical Association (hereinafter the AMA) contributed to this war? It has not. The AMA has maintained a strange, steady silence about the

3

pollution of our food, drugs, and cosmetics with carcinogens. The AMA has remained silent about the non-performance of the FDA and the USDA.

The AMA was founded in 1847 according to a description in "The encyclopedia of Associations." [5] It is an organization that disseminates scientific information to members and the public. It informs members on significant medical and health legislation at state and national levels. It represents the profession before Congress and governmental agencies.

There also is "The American Medical Association Auxiliary," founded in 1922, the members are physicians' wives. It works to meet community needs. It works with the AMA to promote sound health legislation, conducts public education programs. It has interviews with legislators involved in health matters, sponsors a shape up for life campaign to promote good health.

Neither of these august organizations has spoken out to protest the chemicalization of our food supply. The only real cure for cancer is prevention. Why has so very little been said or done by these two organizations to inform people how to prevent cancer?

The Fourth Amendment of the Constitution states "The people have the right to be secure in their persons."

As a people we have not only a cancer plague, we have cancer phobia. We are phobic for a reason. We watch our relatives, friends, neighbors; business acquaintances suffer and die. How can we feel secure in our persons?

How? We know that the FDA suppresses information about dangerous additives in our food. We know that our air is polluted. We know that laws about food additives are not enforced. We know that agribusiness is unrestrained. We know that we live in a cancer culture. How can we feel "secure" in our persons?

1. "At highest Risk", Christopher Norwood, McGraw Hill, New York NY.
2. "The Chemical Feast", The Nader Report, by James S. Turner, Grossman Publishers, 125a East 19th St., New York, NY.
3. "The Chemical Feast."
4. "The Chemical Feast."
5. *Encyclopedia of Associations*, Gale Research, Inc., Detroit, MI.

CHAPTER TWO

The Color Of Cancer

The color of cancer is green. It is big business for the medical establishment. Pharmaceutical companies have rising profit margins, hospitals are busy. It costs the average American between $15,000 and $20,000 to die of cancer.

The chemical cartels that manufacture carcinogenic additives for food know that cancer is green. So do the pesticide companies.

Cancer is basically green, but it also comes in a rainbow of colors. Our food, drugs, and cosmetics are pretty. They are pretty from artificial food colors like yellow, red, blue, and violet to name a few. In 1856, Sir William Henry Perkins synthesized the color mauve from coal tar oil. Synthetic dyes replaced the vegetable and mineral compounds of almost nineteen centuries. The basic compounds of coal tar are triatemylmethane, Azo, indigo, and xanthene. Coal tar is carcinogenic. The development of artificial colors has injured the human race.

What is a color additive? This is a term used to describe a dye, pigment, or other substance capable of coloring a food, drug, or cosmetic or any part of the human body.

We must free the food economy from the use of artificial colors. Artificial colors should be given zero tolerance. Linus Pauling when asked what amount of a compound is needed to sensitize in the human body replied "a single molecule."

The Color Additive Act was passed in 1960. It has not been enforced. Food colors are as frivolous as they are dangerous. They add no nutritional value. They are used solely for cosmetic reasons. In France seven food colors are used. In the U.S.A. seven hundred food colors are used. Consumers have assumed these colors are safe because labels state "U.S. certified artificial color." This is a misleading label.

"Certified" does not mean the color was certified for safety. "Certified" means simply that the color meets government standards that allow a percentage of impurities. By this practice, the government does not have to prove the colors are unsafe. They put the burden on industry according to a law the FDA has not enforced.

The Color Amendment of 1960 has not solved the question of safety in artificial colors. This law has a "permanent part" and a "temporary part." The permanent part called for the testing of colors to prove them safe before they could be added to food.

The temporary part allowed "a provisional listing." This allowed use of the colors pending completion of the scientific investigation needed as a basis for making a determination about their safety. This is just another dodge from doing what must be done to protect consumers.

Not only are artificial colors carcinogenic, they are suspect of causing hyperactivity in children. Dr. Benjamin Feingold structured a nutritional program for hyperactivity in children. This diet eliminated all artificial colors. This diet not only calmed children; it cured an eye condition called nystagmus.

One food processor claims that artificial colors are necessary. Kraft's Consumer Affairs Department published a leaflet and mentioned "color enhancers." The claim is made that "foods must have characteristic and attractive colors." If during the processing, the original color is changed, coloring agents will restore it. About 90 percent of these coloring agents are scientifically produced and about 10 percent are derived from plants. No mention is made in this leaflet about the sources of these "scientifically produced" coloring agents. No proof is offered of their safety.

The FDA printed a booklet called "A Primer on Food Additives." In this publication is a statement "Many of the rich appealing colors we take for granted in today's processed foods are due to the use of color additives." Then a claim is made, "According to the color Additive Amendments of 1960, such food dyes must be safe." Dr. George Pauli, a consumer safety officer with FDA's Division of Food and Color Additives says "These are substances that are so widely known and the information about them is so widely distributed that there is little question about their safety." Other officers of the FDA do

6

not agree with Dr. Pauli. In June of 1985, the FDA found that six colors found in food, drugs, and cosmetics caused cancer in laboratory animals. President Reagan transferred the decision about banning these colors from FDA to the Department of Health and Human Services (herein called HHS). The HHS Secretary Margaret Heckler refused to ban the dyes and offered no reason why the ban was denied.This was a case in which, after years of study and delay, the FDA made a decision to protect the consumer. Unfortunately, it was not allowed to act on this decision. Rep. Ted Weiss, D., N.H. said, "HHS has blatantly violated federal law in failing to ban six potentially hazardous dyes." He also remarked "this has undermined FDA's ability to protect the health and safety of the American public.Artificial colors pollute our food. They are in toothpaste, chewing gum, cough syrup, prescription pills, lipstick, rouge, and patent medicines. The World Health Organization (hereinafter W.H.O.) has questioned the safety of these pervasive artificial colors. Let's examine a few of the many colors.

F.D. and C. blue No. 1
Like other colors, it is a coal tar derivative. It can cause allergy reactions. When injected into laboratory rats, it produced malignant tumors at the site of injection. The rats died in vain– it is still used. It is found in ice cream, soda pop, cereals, candy, puddings, and other foods.

F.D. and C. blue No. 2 indigo carmine.
This contains sulfate or sodium chloride. The WHO said it did not meet requirements for food use, but it remains on FDA's provisional use. It is found in soda pop, candy, cereal, dry drink powders.

F.D. and C. violet No. 1
When this dye was found to cause cancer in half the rats by a Canadian study in 1962, our FDA did not ban it. It was studied. It was used on dogs. In 1971, it was decided to continue the studies. Finally, in 1973 it was banned. This carcinogenic food color remained in our food for eleven years after its danger was discovered. It is still used to stamp meats.

F.D. and C. green No. 1
It was found to be harmful by the W.H.O. It was not used very much and was discontinued.

7

FD and C. green No. 2

This produced tumors at the site of injection under the skin of laboratory rats.

FD and C. green No. 3

This is a sensitizer for allergy victims. It caused malignant tumors at the site of injection in laboratory rats. It is used in cereals, candy mint flavored jelly, gelatin.

FD and C. yellow No. 5 tartrazine

This is another coal tar derivative. When the FDA wanted to list this color with a maximum use of 300 ppm in food, when the color industry objected, the FDA listed it permanently as a color additive with no restrictions.

It can cause life threatening asthma symptoms for allergy sensitive patients. It is used in antihistamines, oral decongestants and in 60 percent of over the counter drugs.

Red dye No. 3 erythrosine

This can interfere with neurotransmitters in the brain. It caused thyroid tumors in rats. It is used in maraschino cherries, sherberts, ice cream, and candy.

The artificial colors must be removed from our food supply and never reintroduced.

While the death rates climb, cancer has spawned a multibillion-dollar industry. Statistics on the situation are proof. In 1971, President Richard Nixon declared war on cancer.

President Nixon signed the National Cancer Act at the White House two days before Christmas of 1971. He called this act "A Christmas present to the nation." He promised "The same kind of concentrated effort that split the atom and took man to the moon."

Now, twenty years and twenty-two million dollars later, cancer claims more lives than before. It is this nation's second leading cause of death and is expected to pass heart disease and become the leading cause of death by the year 2,000.

In 1971, this nation spent two hundred thirty million dollars on cancer. There were 336,000 deaths from this dreaded disease. In 1985, the spending climbed to one billion two hundred million dollars. The deaths climbed to 461,000. By 1991, the spending for the war on cancer reached two billion dollars. The death rate soared to 515,000 that year.

In the last two decades, cancer has increased fifteen percent. The death rates from cancer of the lungs, breast, prostate, and digestive organs have barely changed.

Doctors laboratories research organizations have an ever-escalating income over the years. The cancer industry is Big Business. In 1989, the Cancer Society released its annual report. It showed more than $707 million in stocks, bonds, certificates of deposit, real estate and other assets.

Drug companies have rising profits. In 1990, the profits from cancer drug sales were 1.3 billion dollars. In 1987, the Sloan Kettering Cancer Center in New York had 130 million dollars in security investments. This center does virtually no research into the new therapies for cancer – anyone interested in this situation should read "The Cancer Industry" by Ralph W. Moss, a former Sloan Kettering staff member.

Another book has been published about the problem. "Health Research Charities – The Politics of Fear" reveals how cancer charities have become political lobbies.

The war on cancer has been a failure because it has not stressed prevention. When the medical establishment fought diseases like tuberculosis, malaria, polio, typhus, is stressed prevention.

The only strategy of prevention of cancer has been the crusade against smoking. There has been no large-scale effort to end the pollution of our food, drugs, air, and water. You can stop smoking, but you cannot stop eating. Until this pollution is ended, the war on cancer will fail and the color of cancer will remain green.

CHAPTER THREE

Those Awful Additives

What is an additive? The Food Protection Committee's definition is: "A food additive is a substance or mixture of substances, other than a basic foodstuff, which is present in food as a result of production, processing, storage, or packaging." [6]

There are direct and indirect additives, indirect (or incidental) additives are chemicals, sprayed as insecticides, which leave residues in the food. There are also growth regulators used to increase fruit or vegetable size. Another group of incidental additives is the animal growth stimulants, tranquilizers, and antibiotics used on cattle, sheep, and poultry. Farmers use more antibiotics than doctors.

There is non-disclosure of incidental additives. The Kefauver-Harris Drug Amendments of 1962 made an exemption to the Delaney Amendment, it said drugs or chemicals could be added to animal feeds.

Is there a difference between an additive and an ingredient? The Random House Dictionary defines a food additive as "a substance added directly to food during processing, for preservation, coloring, or stabilization. The same dictionary defines ingredient as "something that enters as an element in a mixture." Examples are given: Flour, eggs, sugar are ingredients in a cake. A second definition states an ingredient is "a constituent element of anything– a component."

A leaflet printed by Oscar Mayer Company Consumer Relations Department claims that "in meat processing the words additive and ingredient are interchangeable." [7]

In an effort to make additives acceptable the claim is made that "all natural foods are chemical as produced by nature." [8] This leaflet closes with the remark that "on the basis of preceding examples one could define the term additive as a minor ingredient added to the major ingredient to achieve a specific desired effect."[9]

I find this verbal hocus pocus to be unacceptable. An additive is not an ingredient. It is added to the basic foodstuff. The question is why? And the next question is what precautions should be taken before an additive is used?

Additives are used to prevent spoilage. Such additives are called preservatives. They are supposed to prevent deterioration and rancidity.Some additives are used as flavor enhancers, some as emulsifiers to maintain consistency. There are ripeners and bleaching agents. Additives used to prevent molds are called fungicides. Pesticides are used to prevent infestation by insects. Food technology in America is becoming dependent on chemical additives.Despite the rationalizations, it is difficult to believe that such dependency is necessary. Why use MSG (Monosodium Glutamate) as a flavor enhancer? There are herbs that are natural flavor enhancers: Garlic, sesame, cumin, coriander, thyme are flavor enhancers.Why use chemical coloring agents when there are natural colors like carmine, annato, caramel, tumeric, xanthophyll, chlorophyllin, beet juice, carotene?

The sun is a growth regulator. Why use anti-oxidants like BHA, BHT, and Propyl Galiate? Their purpose is to increase shelf life. Longer shelf life for a product is not a reason to use chemicals that harm people's health.

What precautions should be taken before an additive is used? Questions should be asked: Will the additives create a toxic condition? Will it break down or be stored in fatty tissue, bones, and the nervous system? How will it effect sick people, the elderly, pregnant women, diabetics, people with allergies? Is it synergistic? Will it combine with another additive to do harm? Such questions should be answered as a precaution against using dangerous additives. To fail to do so violates a provision of the Delaney Amendment– "Manufacturers must show proof of a reasonable certainty that no harm will result from the proposed use of an additive."

There are over six thousand additives in our food. Rules supposed to regulate them are not logical. The FDA requires some to be on labels. Others are exempt. The public has no access to FDA studies on the toxic properties of additives. Scientific data on additives shared by industry and the USDA is not in the public domain.

Additives, which have been proven dangerous often, remain in the food. An example is carrageenan. This is used in salad dressing, cheese, sherbert, and ice cream. It is used in vinegar, wine, and beer to control foam. Carrageenan was used on laboratory animals and induced fatal ulcerative colitis. When fed to guinea pigs, it caused collagen granuloma. It is used in infant formula powder!

Let's examine DEP (diethyl pyrocarbonate). This is tasteless. It is used in beer, wine, malt liquor, and it is a co-carcinogen (when combined with other compounds becomes carcinogenic). It reacts with ammonia to form urethane, an established carcinogen. Once Urethane is formed in food, it stays there. It can break down and form intermediate products, one of which is diethyl carbonate. When this was injected into hamsters it showed teratogenicity. DEP was banned in Sweden in 1971, because research confirmed it as a carcinogen. It is not banned in the U.S.A. and there is not even a requirement that it be listed on the label.

Benzoic Acid is a chemical preservative on the GRAS list. It is used in margarine, codfish, pickles, jelly, jam, soft drinks, ice cream, candy, and gum. It was tested in Soviet Russia on mice for eight months and on rats for eighteen months. The laboratory animals became thin and evidence emerged that it is a co-carcinogen. Its use was restricted.

Later Soviet tests showed more adverse effects. The animal's growth and survival rates were impaired. When it was combined with sodium bisulfate the toxic effect was greater. It was found to be toxic to humans, causing irritation to the skin and mucous membranes. The USSR's Food Hygiene Department of the Ministry of Health accepted these findings and placed tighter restrictions on the use of benzoate and sulfites in preservatives.

One of the additives now in use, which has been intentionally kept off the list of additives that must be put on labels, is BVO. Brominated Vegetable Oils are used in bakery products, soft drinks, ice cream, and other frill foods as a stabilizing agent. In order to produce BVO, edible oils are saturated with a toxic substance: Bromine. This is stored in human tissue.

In 1967, officials in Belgium stated that the use of BVO in soft drinks was no longer authorized. Sweden banned it in 1968 in 1969 and 1970, the British Industrial Biological Research Association did experimental work which produced damaging evidence regarding

BVO. When it was fed into the diet of rats at a level of 0.5g it interfered with their metabolism. It produced high fat deposits in their kidneys and hearts. When fed to pigs, it was stored in their spleens with high concentrates in their pancreas, lungs, liver, and heart.

Studies made by the Canadian Food and Drug Directorate showed adverse changes in rats given low levels of BVO for eighty days. They suffered growth retardation, anemia, and enlargement of the heart, kidneys, and spleen. Animals given BVO at a 2.5 feeding level showed arrested testicular development. In January of 1970, the Canadian Minister of Health ordered reduction of its use. In February of 1970, British officials removed BVO from the list of permitted stabilizers and in September of that year announced it would no longer be permitted in food or drink.

In the wake of these findings, what happened in the U.S.A.? In 1970, Charles Edwards, the FDA Commissioner, said "The Canadian and British studies were inconclusive." He allowed American food and beverage processors to continue using BVO pending further study.

Not everyone is as casual as Charles Edwards was about dangerous additives. Senator Abraham Ribicoff said, "The American people have generally assumed that new food additives have been tested by the government and licensed as safe. This proves to be anything but the case." Dr. Samuel S. Epstein of the Children's Cancer Research Foundation and the Harvard Medical School believes consumer protection laws should involve testing the safety of food additives before allowing them to be used.

An example of a dangerous additive that was used without precaution is cyclamate. The cyclamates were removed from beverages years after it was proven they caused liver cancer in laboratory animals. Dr. Jacqueline Verrett, the Biochemist whose testimony had them banned, laid her job on the line when she spoke out. Her book, "Eating may be dangerous to your health" was quickly suppressed.

What happened with MSG? Monosodium Glutamate. Gerber and Heinz were adding MSG to baby food. Herbert L. Ley, then Commissioner of FDA tried to justify its usage. He was challenged by Ralph Nader's Research Group. Jim Turner, Head of this group said, "Clearly MSG should not be used in baby food– and should have been removed as soon as doubts were raised about its safety."

MSG was removed from baby food five months after reports were

13

made that it caused brain damage in laboratory mice. It was removed only because of public pressure after Nader's group testified before a Senate Hearing on its danger. It was not removed because the FDA was conscientiously doing its job.

The United States Department of Agriculture allows nitrite in excessive levels. It is in bacon, ham, luncheon meats, and sausage.

In 1971, a scientist at USDA's Eastern Research Laboratory at Wyndmore, PA, found dimethylnitrosamine (DNM) at 80 ppb in sample hotdogs from a supermarket. A press release about this never left the USDA. Then, three months later, the USDA announced this Pennsylvania discovery, but said new samples proved negative.

The FDA and the USDA operate on the theory that a little dose of carcinogen will not hurt you. They really believe they can establish a "safe" level of carcinogens. The Surgeon General asked a committee of eight scientists to evaluate carcinogens in 1970. They stated, "It is impossible to establish any absolutely safe level of exposure to a carcinogen for man."

This committee also said, "The National Academy of Sciences National Research Council Food Protection Committee's 'safe' level has absolutely no validity and displays a lack of understanding of the irreversible and delayed toxic effects which occur in carcinogenesis."

Herbicides are an example of incidental additives. Chlorophenoxy chemicals are dangerous herbicides. They enter the roots of plants in thirty minutes and within two hours are in the stem and leaves.

Chlordacetamides kiss grass weeds. Naphthalene acetamide is a spray used on plants. These additives are called agrochemical. They are health hazards.

One of the most dangerous direct additives was Alar. This chemical was used to speed the ripening process of apples. It seeped into apple juice and applesauce. It was a known carcinogen.

Not until there was a public outcry, did Uniroyal, the manufacturer of Alar, stop selling this chemical. The Environmental Protection Agency (EPA) finally banned the use of Alar on all food.

After the Alar scandal, the National Academy of Science, using EPA data, made a list of foods which could be a threat to public health if sprayed with chemicals at the maximum amount. The foods, which are high risk when toxic agrochemical is used, are Tomatoes, potatoes, oranges, lettuce, apples, peaches, wheat, soybeans, carrots, corn, and grapes.

14

Beef and pork can be a threat because pesticides used on animal feed can accumulate in animal tissues. Chicken is often contaminated. Des Diethylstilbestrol (DES) is still used on chicken, even though it is legally banned.

Oranges are a good source of Vitamin C. Actually, Brussels sprouts have 70 percent more Vitamin C than do oranges. Still, oranges are, under normal circumstances, a healthy food. But we do not have a "normal" food supply in the U.S. For example, let us examine the California orange supply. The most commonly used insecticide on oranges is dimethoate. It is used to control thrips— insects that scar the peel but do not harm the inside of the fruit. It is very toxic. However, the orange co-operatives, which operate under federal rules, ban scarred fruit from the marketplace. By joint agreement, they have no such agreement to ban fruits contaminated with Dimethoate. A very good fruit— the orange— has been turned into a toxic, unhealthy food.

Over sixty of the more than 300 ingredients in pesticides are human carcinogens. Farmers should stop their dependence on chemicals. They should rotate their crops. They should control pests with natural predators like ladybugs. The EPA is asleep at the wheel and the health of the American consumer suffers.

Before modern chemicals were developed, how did farmers and home gardeners rid their crops of insects? How did people control pests before chemical pesticides and herbicides were available? Long ago there were no sprays. Yet, crops of vegetables and fruits survived.

There were beneficial insects that ate the unwanted pests. There was a system of companion planting. Strong odored plants, like garlic and hot peppers growing close to crop plantings, kept bugs away. Nutrient-rich garden soil helped plants that had been chewed by these pests to survive.

Leo Van Meer, a garden columnist, described his mother's techniques. She saved soapy dish water in wood barrels. Then he, as a boy, carried it to the garden and, with a tin dipper, sloshed it on the bug-infested plants. Sometimes his mother made concoctions of garlic and peppers to kill the pests. Sometimes Fels Naphtha soap, soaked in a pan of water was used. If pesticides or chemicals dangerous to humans can be made in large vats, so can non-toxic pesticides made in large quantities. There has to be a commitment from the companies that sell pesticides. These businesses have to study organic

15

procedures.

6. "Chemical and Biological hazards in Food," Iowa State University Press, page 3, Ames, Iowa.
7. Oscar Mayer Consumer Relations Pamphlet, Oscar Mayer, Inc., PO Box 7188, Madison, Wisconsin 53707.
8. Ibid.
9. Ibid.

CHAPTER FOUR

Deadly Drugs

Anyone who assumes that the drug company executives have a social conscience is naïve and unrealistic. The criteria these people use when introducing a new drug should be: Is it safe? Is it effective? The question asked: Is it profitable?

Take the case of the drug Chloromycetin. By June of 1952 the F. D. A. withdrew certification because a national survey showed 177 cases of blood disorders like leukemia and hypoplastic anemia. Parke Davis knew the statistics.

When Chloromycetin came on the market, deaths from aplastic anemia climbed, and when it was withdrawn, deaths dropped. When it was re-introduced, deaths climbed.

Did Parke Davis comply willingly when the F. D. A. withdrew certification? Chloromycetin accounted for one third of this company's profits[1]. No, this company insisted the drug was safe, and pressured doctors to prescribe it. The company ran ads in medical journals which claimed the drug was effective for everything from the common cold to dermatological conditions.

A mild disclaimer said serious blood disorders from it were rare and that blood studies were needed when a patient was given the drug for prolonged use.

Sales climbed. Although 70% of the aplastic anemia cases from this drug were fatal, ads proclaimed "children really like the taste of this custard flavored preparation."[2]

An Italian ad for Chloromycetin said, "The preparation has been tolerated well by both adults and infants. In the few cases in which reactions have occurred, they have been generally limited to slight nausea or diarrhea and their severity rarely requires suspension of

17

treatment."[3]

There was no mention of the fatal blood diseases. The greed was total. Money is more important than human life. This attitude is reflected by other drug companies and the Pharmaceutical Manufacturers Association.

The Thalidomide tragedy in England and Germany was avoided in the U. S. A. because of the efforts of Dr. Frances D. Kelsey. She was with the Division of New Drugs of the F. D. A.

Despite pressure from the William S. Merrell Company to approve the drug, she refused to give approval for distribution. As the evidence of its deadly effects was mounting and its dangers were confirmed, Merrell withdrew its application.

The results of the tragedy proved the glaring necessity to control advertising for a new drug and to demand that a drug company prove its safety.

After this incident, the pharmaceutical Manufacturers Association was no longer able to make false claims so freely. In 1962, Congress passed amendments requiring F. D. A. inspection for new drugs.

North Carolina Congressman L. H. Fountain insisted on reforms in the way new drugs were inspected and improved. Thanks to his committee, the efforts of F. D. A. Commissioner Dr. Herbert Ley to remove dangerous drugs from the market were successful.

Congressman Ley insisted the F. D. A. curtail the abuses the pharmaceutical industry had perpetrated on consumers. He did not want consumers used as guinea pigs. He did not want Americans to live in a drugged society.

Dr. Richard Burack, an Affiliate in Pharmacology at Harvard Medical School, wrote a book, "The New Handbook of Prescription Drugs". He was dismayed that the drug industry spent large sums of money on advertisements in medical journals.

Dr. Burack noted that many of the ads were false and misleading. He believed that persons who were hospitalized from side effects were victims of the profit-making mentality of drug companies.

Dr. Burack advocated the use of generic names for drugs. He thought it inexcusable that executives of the F. D. A. were so obsequious to the drug companies. The agency which is supposed to protect the consumers helps to victimize them.

It is bad enough that some drugs are, in their own chemical make-up, carcinogens. Worse yet, is the danger that many drugs contain

18

Amines that can be nitrosated in the stomach. Over-the-counter and prescription drugs can produce Nitrosamines when taken for a long time.

Some of the drugs that can yield nitros derivatives are: Aminopyrine, Methadone, Disfiram - - Antabuse, Tolazamide. It was thought that adding Vitamin C to the drug formula would reduce Nitrosamine yields.

But this did not prevent nitrosation. It would be better if the drug industry could develop drugs without amines. That is expecting too much of an industry that shows no remorse for lives already lost to its practice of putting lethal drugs on the market.

Drug companies are still selling drugs which are known carcinogens. Grisefulvin, which is used for the minor complaint of athlete's foot, is carcinogenic. We need a law requiring testing for carcinogenicity before a drug is allowed on the market.

The drug industry lacks a conscience. How was D. E. S. handled? Diethylstibesterol is a synthetic estrogen. It can cause cancer. This was known as long ago as the 1940's. Not until 1959 did the F. D. A. decide to suspend new drug applications for its use in animal feeds.

In 1968, the F. D. A. discovered evidence that D. E. S. could cause cancer in daughters of women who had taken it. This discovery led in 1971 to the F. D. A. advising doctors to use caution about giving D. E. S. to pregnant women.

How did the drug company that produced D. E. S. show concern? Eli Lilly and Co. claimed that the writings of authorities in enducrinology had "Demonstrated that Stilbesterol is safe as administered to human beings.

Dr. Carney claimed that an article in the "Journal of the American Medical Association" had concluded there was "No danger of cancer production from estrogen treatment." His claim was proven false when daughters of women who had taken the drug during pregnancy had to be treated for vaginal cancer.

What of the sanctity of human life? It is not a consideration. Drug companies have ways of convincing doctors to use their products.

Doctors are taking cash perks from drug companies. These doctors are more likely to ask their hospital to add a new drug to its official medication list than doctors who do not take perks.

A study of this was made by Dr. Mary Margaret Chren of Case

19

Western Reserve University in Cleveland, Ohio. Dr. Chren and Dr. Charles Landefeld surveyed forty doctors who made 55 consecutive requests for drugs to be added to the university hospital's formulary.

Dr. Chren compared responses from 80 hospital doctors selected at random. The doctors who made requests were seven times more likely to have received money from a company for research, lectures, or going to dinners and symposiums.

Doctors requesting use of new drugs were 2½ times more likely to have accepted funds from companies whose drugs they had requested than from other drug companies.

Doctors who made such requests were four times more likely to have met with drug company agents than doctors who did not make requests.

Doctors have taken, as a routine, millions of dollars each year in perks like cash, dinners, vacations, and prizes from drug companies. Consumer groups should protest this long and loud. The practice of such gift taking has been condemned by the A. M. A. but continues.

The safety and effectiveness of a new drug should indicate its acceptance. It should not be recommended to a hospital because a doctor had a vacation at the expense of a drug company.

The most commonly prescribed drugs in the U. S. A. are tranquilizers. The next most commonly used drugs are female hormones. These are not just used on humans. They are used in animal feeds to stimulate growth in cattle, hogs and poultry.

Estrogens used in contraceptives have become big business. Investigations into possible hazards of such pills have been inadequate. The use of contraceptive pills is the world's largest use of uncontrolled drugs which could prove to be carcinogenic.

The fact is that estrogen and other female sex hormones may have been proven to be carcinogenic. Animal experiments have suggested that such hormones involve risk of liver tumors and cancer of the breast and cervix. Premarin has resulted in a virtual epidemic of uterine cancer.

D. E. S. is a synthetic chemical which acts like an estrogen. It has given evidence of causing breast cancer and vaginal cancer in the daughters of women who used it. This is still used in feed for cattle and lambs!

The deaths of innocent people from known carcinogens in their food and drugs are murders. These carcinogens are in our food and drug supply illegally. They are there because the Delaney Amendment has not been enforced.

Citizens should not have to research and study these carcinogens. But we must do so. People in government agencies are paid to learn about them and ban the ones found dangerous. At present, consumers take these carcinogens into their systems without informed consent.

A skull and crossbones should be on the label of every drug which is carcinogenic. People have a moral as well as a legal right to know the risk before taking any life-threatening substance.

The deliberate poisoning of our food, drugs, cosmetics from a motive of greed has resulted in a self-destructive type of fatalism. This pollution has consumers remarking, "Everything I eat or drink is bad for me, so I will just ignore the risk and consume it." This attitude is good for the chemical industry and agribusiness for whom it is business as usual.

It is welcomed by government bureaucrats whose sins of omission and commission brought the situation into existence. Such as attitude will not bring changes needed to help America win the war on cancer.

A classical example of how a carcinogenic drug can be easily obtained is the way Tylenol (Generic name) has been handled. Tylenol is Acetaminophen, a chemical so powerful that a human fetus is at risk when a large dose of it crosses into fetal circulation.

Tylenol and alcohol can be a deadly combination. The "Journal of the American Medical Association" stated in 1980, "There is continuing evidence that Acetaminophen may not be as safe as it seems. Patients should be warned that the co-administration of alcohol and Acetaminophen at least in high therapeutic doses may be harmful."

Tylenol is advertised as an alternative to aspirin. People take it in similar doses. This is dangerous. According to Dr. Mark Katz, Associate Director of Emergency Services at Madison General Hospital, "Tylenol is likely to cause more deaths than just about any drug in your medicine cabinet."

This drug is toxic in a silent way. The signs of over dosage do not appear for three or four days and by then liver damage is irreversible. Dr. Katz sees an over dosage of Tylenol once a week and thinks it is unfortunate there will be more deaths before this drug is either banned or sold by prescription only.

Adults taking daily doses of Acetaminophen on a long term basis

21

have increased risk of kidney disease. A study in Germany revealed this.

A study was conducted by Dale P. Sandler at The National Institute of Environmental Health Sciences in Research Triangle Park, North Carolina. Her team had telephone interviews with 554 adults diagnosed with kidney disease and 516 matched controls. They were questioned about the use of analgesics.

Those who used Acetaminophen had a three fold risk of kidney disease according to the report in "The New England Journal of Medicine.

Pediatricians have theorized that normal doses of Acetaminophen can produce severe toxic effects on kidneys of children. Warning labels of this product are not sufficient. It should be banned. It is a carcinogen.

American consumers have assumed that prescriptions and non-prescription drugs on the market have been honestly and thoroughly tested. There is a misconduct in drug research.

According to the May, 1989 "Journal of the American Medical Association", the F. D. A. should take stronger action to weed out incompetent or dishonest researchers.

This is the opinion of Martin F. Shapiro of the University of California and Robert P. Charrow, formerly with the Department of Human Services in Washington, D. C.

When researchers are hired by drug companies to study experimental drugs, the F. D. A. sends investigators to study the laboratory records. These records from June, 1977 to April, 1988 were studied by Shapiro and Charrow. Their audit found serious deficiencies like failure to obtain informed consent from patients in about 12% before 1985. Then down to 7%.

Although it seems incredible, every year four hundred thousand Americans die of Iatrogenic (doctor caused) illness. No, doctors are not deliberately killing their patients. However, they are not doing what needs to be done to prevent these unnecessary deaths. They are not doing their homework. They do not study the possible lethal side effects of new deadly drugs.

The problem has several facets. Too many doctors are drug oriented. They prescribe drugs for chronic conditions, which could be treated with safer more effective methods like hydrotherapy, acupuncture, and a nutrition program.

22

This situation benefits the drug cartels whose purpose is to make money. Drug cartels spend millions of dollars promoting their wares. If they warn consumers about sickening, even lethal side effects of drugs, the profit margin will not rise.

How do doctors obtain information on the powerful drugs that they so blithely prescribe? Do they do independent research on the chemical components of the drug? Do they strive to ascertain whether the drug could harm a pregnant woman, a fetus, an elderly patient, and an allergy patient? How much time do they spend in an effort to learn the side effects? Are they zealous about learning if the drug could conflict with other drugs and cause toxic drug interaction?

Four hundred thousand deaths every year indicate that there are too many doctors who prescribe drugs about which they know very little or nothing at all. How do doctors learn about new drugs?

Doctors depend on the detail man employed by the drug company for whom he is selling the drug. He is not going to lose a sale by mentioning that a specific drug can cause aplastic anemia, a fatal blood disorder for which there is no cure. Such drugs are on the market today.

To become knowledgeable, a consumer can read about drugs. At the end of the Chapter I list books about commonly used prescription and non-prescription pills. There is a publication called The Physician's Desk Reference. This is not printed independently by people concerned with the health and safety of consumers. Drug companies pay the publisher to list their products.

The Trade Association for Drug Companies is the Pharmaceutical Manufacturer's Association. Its purpose is to keep drug prices high and promote ineffective drugs. It is of no interest to them if drugs are dangerous, even lethal. Unrestrained by the FDA's failure to enforce the Delaney Amendment, they have lied to, deceived and endangered American consumers. A letter to this Association would get no results. They are ruthless. All they understand is profit margins. They would understand a boycott of their products, resulting in lost money.

Who are these giant drug companies that keep sick people at highest risk of toxic side effects? Who are these drug companies that flout the law of the land? You can obtain their names in the reference room at your public library. Ask for "The National Directory-General Information". It is published in Bothell, Wash. 98011.

A partial list:

Upjohn, Upjohn – Fine Chemical Division, 410 Sackett Point Rd., North Haven, CT 06423.

Eli Lilly Co. Lilly Corporate Center, Indianapolis, IN 46285.

Abbot Laboratories. 1 Abbot Park Dr., IL 60064. Lederle Laboratories, 401 N. Middleton Rd., Pearl River, NH 10965.

Before you conclude I am judging too harshly, allow me to describe some of the side effects of commonly used drugs. These are drugs on the market that can cause: Ulcerative Colitis, heart attack, cancer, severe bone marrow depression, damage to lungs, liver, kidney-jaundice, reduced levels of red and white blood cells, aplastic anemia, high blood pressure, asthma, psychotic reactions, increased cholesterol, anaphylaxis, Parkinson-like diseases, etc. There are cures that can kill.

The FDA has withheld information about this situation. They have ignored doctors' reports on adverse side effects. According to the General Accounting Office (hereinafter GAO), the FDA has not fulfilled its responsibilities to regulate drugs. The FDA has harassed doctors who complained that certain drugs should be on non-approval status.

The AMA does not show any interest in efforts to test drugs for safety or efficacy. This organization has been uninterested in drug safety. If a drug is toxic or habit forming– so what? Millions of people are prescribed medicine every week and there are no restraints on the doctors' use of drugs, which have not been proven safe.

There are two drug abuse problems in America. The abuse of illegal drugs and the abuse of prescription and patent drugs. The problem of drug abuse of legal pills is critical in the elderly. More than half of the deaths from side effects of prescription drugs are in over 60 age group. The elderly are only 17 percent of the population.

What can a person do? When given a prescription, ask the doctor about possible side effects– if his answers are evasive or inadequate, go to the reference room of your library, and look up the drug in one of the books I list.

Better yet! Learn about healing therapies that do not involve drugs– for example, you have sinus problems. Instead of buying a decongestant pill– put your teakettle on and breathe the steam or use a vaporizer. If you have arthritis which is chronic– try the water exercises illustrated in a book called "Pain free arthritis by Dvera Berson– Simon and Schuster, New York, New York. This book is a magnificent breakthrough on a non-toxic therapy for arthritis. Gentle stretching exercises in room temperature water can stop symptoms. People with arthritis should swim at least three times a week.

The first consideration when diagnosed for sickness should be *diet.* Arthritis victims should learn the proper nutrition for this chronic disease. It is like lupus and multiple sclerosis, a disease of the immune system. Since sugar devastates the immune system, sugar is the first "food" to *GO!*

The drugs prescribed for arthritis are among the deadliest. Cytoxan and Imuran can cause cancer. Feldene is a disaster. It should never be taken by anyone on blood thinners. Pfizer has 77 wrongful death lawsuits over Feldene. Petitions were sent by senior citizens' group to the FDA to remove Feldene from the market. The FDA ignored them.

This entire situation reminds me of a story I heard years ago. A farmer called a veterinarian to come and help his sick cow. The veterinarian traveled out to the farm and prescribed medicine. A few weeks later the farmer was in town and met the veterinarian who inquired about the health of the cow. The farmer replied, "The cow is cured of her sickness, but is dead of the medicine."

Actually, there are medicines that are non chemical and require no prescription. The whole field of homeopathic medicine so popular in England waits to be explored. Herbs have marvelous healing qualities. Hippocrates, the father of medicine, used herbs. Ancient doctors relied on herbs. Their big advantage is that they are not processed in a laboratory, into a pill which carcinogenic artificial colors. Some dedicated modern doctors are learning about and using herbs.

Modern antibiotics were developed from molds. Digitalis, a heart drug, is derived from foxglove. Garlic lowers blood pressure. The Journal of the National Cancer Institute published a report that garlic can reduce the risk of stomach cancer. Ginger is good for arthritis and can reduce cholesterol. There are 12 herbs that have anti-tumor properties.

Herbs are medicine and cannot be taken without knowledge of their possible side effects. If you want to take herbs consult a doctor who knows about them. Ginger is safe. No one is in the cemetery from the side effects of ginger ale or ginger bread. Blackberry is still being studied because it contains tannin, which may contribute to stomach cancer. A book with information on herbs is called "The Healing Herbs"– the ultimate guide to the curative power of nature's medicine" by Michael Castleman, Rodale Press, 33 East Minor St., Emmals, PA 18098.

1. "The Essential Guide to Prescription Drugs." James W. Longman, Harper & Row Publishers, Inc., 10 East 53rd St., New York, NY 10022.
2. The Essential Guide to Generic Drugs", M. Lawrence Lieberman, R. Pu, Harper and Row, New York.
3. Children's' Medicine, Ann and James Kepler with Ira Salafsky, M.D.
4. Contemporary Books, Inc., 180 Worth, Michigan Ave., Chicago, IL 60601.
5. Joe Graedon's "The New People's Pharmacy," Joe and Teresa Graedon, Bantam Books, Inc. 666 Fifth Ave., New York, NY 10103.
6. "Worst Pills, Best Pills." The Older Adult's Guide to Drug Induced Death and Illness."
7. Public Citizens' Health Research Group, 2000 "P" St., NW, Suite 700, Washington, DC 20036 by Sidney M. Wolff, Lisa Fugate, Elizabeth P. Hillstrand, Laurie E. Kamimoto.

8. Essential Guide to Non Prescription Drugs, David R. Zimmerman, Harper & Row, New York, NY

The above is a partial list of books available in libraries. Two inexpensive books in paperback are:

"The Prescription Drug Encyclopedia F.C. & A. DEA PCC-46, 103 Clover Green, Peachtree City, Georgia $7.48

"The Pill Book," Gilbert I. Simon Scd., Harold M. Silverman, Pharm D. Bantam Books Dept. MF 13, 414 East Golf Rd., Des Plaines, IL 60016

There are other books– the point is: consumers do not have to take pills that cause damage and are colored by carcinogenic dyes. They can tell their doctor, "I want a white pill." Write the pharmaceutical company and ask why they use carcinogenic dyes? When we speak out, the companies that are in business will listen. Consumers have a right to safe drugs.

Chemical Manufacturers Association, 2501 "M" St. NW, Washington, DC 20037.

Cosmetic Toiletry and Fragrance Association, 1110 Vermont Ave., NW, Suite 800, Washington, DC 20005.

Grocery Manufacturers of America, 1010 Wisconsin Ave., NW, Suite 800, Washington, DC 20007.

National Confectioners Association of the U.S.A., 7900 Westpark Dr., Suite A-320, McLean, VA 22102.

National Food Processors Association, 1401 New York Ave., NW, 4th Floor. Washington, DC 20005.

Snack Food Association, 1711 King St., Suite 1, Alexandria, VA 22314

The names of more trade associations are listed in "The Encyclopedia of Associations." This is available in the reference room of most public libraries. It is published by Gayle Research, Inc., PO Box 441914, Detroit, MI 48244.

CHAPTER FIVE

The Death Of The Innocents

The incidence of cancer in children has increased. Cancer is now second on the list of causes of death in the 3-14 year age bracket. Accidents are number one.

In cancer, cells reproduce in an abnormal way. When they divide they do not produce normal cells. They produce more cancer cells. A normal cell stops growing in response to influences. Cancer cells do not stop growing. Cells can keep growing to form a tumor. When cancer cells cramp normal organs and cut off food supply to them, the cancer kills the patients. What triggers this abnormal cell growth? Viruses? Radiation? Chemicals?

It is believed a virus can cause leukemia. Leukemia kills more children than adults. Factors like genetic abnormalities and chemicals can cause this disease in which useless white blood cells flood the blood stream.

Some experts believe that cancer in children is a congenital malformation or a result of radiation exposure during pregnancy. There are theories that some families are cancer prone. Environmental factors were discounted as important in childhood cancer.

It is hard to accept that childhood cancer is not caused by environmental factors. When a waste site in Pelham Bay, New York became toxic, twelve cases of leukemia were diagnosed in children living near the site.

As the food supply became saturated with carcinogenic additives, cancer in children increased. It is no longer rare. It has increased to such an extent that there are cancer camps for children. St. Jude's

Children's Research Hospital in Memphis, Tennessee engages in research to find methods of extending life for the many children who have cancer. Special programs help children who are terminal. There is the Teddi Project in Rochester, NY, and the Sunshine Foundation in Philadelphia, PA.

The Candlelighters Childhood Cancer Foundation helps children and parents. It publishes a youth newsletter. Its address is:

The Candlelighters Childhood Cancer Foundation
Suite 1011
2025 Eye St. NW
Washington, DC 20006

Children's oncology camps of America is a volunteer agency headed by Dr. Edward S. Baum of Children's Memorial Hospital in Chicago, Illinois. These camps are not places where gloom prevails. Normal fun activities go on at cancer camps. Hiking, fishing, swimming, horseback riding, etc. are enjoyed. A medical station takes care of the young campers' medical needs.

It is a tragic situation that the need for such services is growing. It is important to comfort and help children, but it is urgent to stop the increase in childhood cancer and prevent the suffering that necessitates such efforts. It is sad that children are being counseled to help them try to accept the unacceptable: death at an early age.

The American Pediatric Society is a professional academic society of educators and researchers interested in the study of children and their diseases. The American Academy of Pediatrics is a professional society of medical doctors engaged in the health care and medical treatment of children. Such organizations are working to prevent death at an early age.

The Association for Research of Childhood Cancer– PO Box 251, Buffalo, New York, 14225 is another organization of merit. The members are parents who lost children to various pediatric cancers. They seek to fund the expansion and continuation of research in pediatric cancer centers and to provide seed money for pilot projects in cancer research.

In reading about cancer in children, I was appalled at how easily it is explained away. Simplistic explanations for its causes are given very blandly and environmental factors are airily dismissed with a wave of the hand. Children get cancer because of a family tendency or

29

because of a random error in the distribution of DNA during a phase of cell multiplication. I can accept these premises as causing some of the cancer in children.

I can accept the premise that some children get cancer because mothers had radiation of drugs or hormones during pregnancy. I cannot accept the fact that American children get cancer more than children in other countries– when the aforementioned causes exist in other countries. What is different here in the USA?

Environmental factors differ and regardless of claims by the medical establishment that such factors rarely cause childhood cancer– I am convinced that the environmental factors causing childhood cancer are a very, very, important consideration in any effort to reduce cancer in children.

The devastating impact of this disease on a child cannot be overestimated. The physical pain of treatments like chemotherapy and surgery is matched by the emotional suffering and mental anguish. How does a child, bald from chemotherapy, feel about going to school? How does a child, knowing he or she is dying, feel about being denied a normal life span? How does a child react to being in and out of a hospital like a yo-yo?

If we can do even one thing to stop this devastation we better do it. I have done research every day for over twenty years in the field of nutrition. I am shocked to learn how polluted are the foods that are advertised to appeal to children– a walk through the cereal section of a supermarket is an eye opener.

It has been proven that artificial food colors are carcinogens. They are banned in civilized countries like France, England, and Canada to name a few. Yet, in defiance of the Pure Food Drug and Cosmetic Act, they saturate our food supply. There are in toothpaste, lipstick, and pills. It seems a Herculean chore to find food, drugs, or cosmetics not laced with artificial colors.

Children's food is BIG BUSINESS. Watch a kiddy cartoon show on TV on Saturday morning and study the commercials, candy and cereal, cereal and candy. Not only are such products colored with deadly dyes, they contain additives like BHT, BHA, TBHQ. The commercials are very persuasive. Get a free toy in the box. Join the club– be like the sports stars. Enjoy the delicious taste. The naïve child is convinced. Claims of being fortified with vitamins and minerals are made. They appeal to mothers.

In an effort to get real I hereby submit a list of cereals today that are aimed at our young consumers– and I will mention the few safe cold cereals on the market. "Fruity Pebbles" contain artificial colors, BHA, artificial flavors– General Foods Company, Box P13, White Plains, NY 10625. "Teen Age Mutant Ninja Turtles" cereal with sodium hexametaphosphate, BHT, artificial colors, artificial flavors calls itself "fortified with 6 essential vitamins and iron." Processed at Ralston Purina Company Checkerboard Square, St. Louis, Missouri, 63164.

Ralston "Cookie Crisp" claims "No cholesterol, no tropical oils" contains BHT, glycerin, yellow dye no. 5, yellow dye No. 6 and artificial flavors.

"Lucky Charms" claims to "provide 8 essential vitamins and iron" contain red dye No. 40, blue dyes No. 1 and 2, yellow dye no. 6 and "other color added." Also artificial flavors. General Mills, Minneapolis, MN 55440.

Also from General Mills– "Oatmeal Crisp"– made from whole grain oats, BHT, artificial flavor.

"Fruit Loops" claims "all natural flavors" contains red dye No. 40 and yellow dye No. 6. Kellogg's, Battle Creek, MI, 49016. This is a partial list of cereals– laced with cancer causing additives that are advertised to appeal to children.

Safe cereals include Raisin Bran, Grape Nuts, KIX, Puffed Rice, Special K, Product 19, Kellogg's Raisin Bran.

Children's cereal is a $7 billion dollar industry. There is no concern about what the carcinogenic additives are doing to their children. The American Academy of Pediatrics has advocated a ban on food commercials aimed at children. The doctors warn that the sugar content causes obesity and high cholesterol in children.

Parents must control their children's diets. Children age 1 to 5 eat more snack foods and drink more soda pop than children did ten years ago. Parents should provide healthy snacks: fruit, yogurt, etc., and should monitor the TV their children watch. The TV commercials promote worthless junk foods. They push cereals, which have no value, candy and junk food, snacks.

Our children cannot defend themselves. We have to protect them from the avarice of the food industry and the betrayal of the FDA. Here is a sample of a letter that could be mailed in protest.

To Whom It May Concern:

Please be advised I will no longer buy your product. Through reading I have learned that yellow dye No. 5 is a carcinogen. I have learned that B.H.T. has never been proven safe. I have told my friends about the dangerous additives in your product. I have notified the manager of the store where I shop that I will not buy your product and told him why. There are alternate cereals, which are free of additives, and I will be buying them.

Sincerely,
Mary Smith

There are genetic factors, which cause cancer in children. We cannot control them, but we can curb the environmental factors that are endangering our children. The government has shown no inclination to enforce laws that would protect our children. It is up to us.

In order to protect our children from cancer, we should learn why there is an increase in the incidence of cancer in young people. One of the explanations is the food supply. It is saturated with carcinogens.

Another explanation is the fact that children are being overexposed to radiation. The tissues of children are more responsive to radiation than those of adults. Excessive use of x-rays in children is more dangerous than in adults.

The younger the child, the Greater the sensitivity to radiation. Studies of survivors of Hiroshima and Nagasaki have proven this.

When a fetus is radiated, the damage can be Leukemia or other diseases. Dr. Gilbert W. Beebe of the Clinical Epidemiology Division– National Cancer Institute, in Washington D.C. stated, "It seems certain that irradiation of the embryo or fetus can cause major defects at birth. Among these; small size and diminished intelligence are the most frequent." [1]

Delayed effects from x-rays are found frequently among children. Dr. Joel Gray and other experts at Mayo Clinic are working to develop methods of reducing doses of x-rays used for pediatric diagnosis.

Irradiation of the body can cause leukemia and other malignancy. Cancer and Leukemia from doses of one Rad and 10 Rads cannot be repaired. There is no x-ray exam that exposes only one cancer-prone organ.[3]

Children have been given x-ray treatment around the neck for enlarged tonsils, bronchitis, adenoids, enlargement of the thyroid gland have been used as conditions which require x-ray. As the practice of x-raying children increased, so did cancer of the thyroid gland in children increase.

Dental x-rays involve large doses of radiation. Fluoroscopy in which the x-ray machine operates at a high dose rate involves the greatest radiation risk.

The average dental film runs about 5r and can go to 14r if the dentist does not use filters.[4] A child who has an annual dental checkup that involves x-rays is at risk.

Large doses of radiation may cause infections of the teeth and destruction to the jawbone. Dr. Max Cutler said, "A simple extraction of a tooth following extensive irradiation in the jaw region has been the cause of death in a considerable number of patients."[5]

Bone damage and cancer result from deposits in the bones of radioactive isotopes like Radium, Plutonium, and Strontium. Small amounts of these isotopes can cause destruction of bone. Repeated dental x-rays of children can damage tissues of the gums and cause serious trouble years later.

Radiation therapy for skin conditions is very hazardous for children. It should not be used for acne. The so-called "strawberry" birthmarks usually disappear in a few years. It can take five years, but they usually go away on their own. Parents are advised not to have them removed by radiation except as a last resort. Fifteen or twenty years later, the harm can show up as skin cancer or Leukemia.

Ringworm of the scalp is another childhood problem, which should be treated by other therapies.

To induce bone cancer, doses of 3,000 are needed. But young, growing bone is more sensitive and radiation of 150 r in infants and 300 r in children can disturb bone formation. The younger the child, the greater the sensitivity to radiation. The use of x-rays for diagnosis and treatment has been overdone. Caution has not been used.

Radiation or pregnant women should be done only if urgent. Studies made by some of the children exposed to radiation in the mother's womb during atomic bombing in Japan revealed a high rate of Leukemia.

Other abnormalities of children who were radiated in the womb are: Mongolism, cleft palate, clubfeet, and mental and physical deficiencies. It is very important to consider all alternate methods of diagnosis and treatment for pregnant women. Unborn children, infants, and children should be protected from unnecessary radiation.

In 1907, radiation was used to treat an enlarged thymus in an infant: This was the first time radiation exposure to children has been documented. Not until the 1940's was there any information available that suggested radiation could be a health hazard to children.

Instead of falling into disfavor, radiation was increasingly used on young patients. Children are very susceptible to the hazard of radiation exposure. Their tissues are more responsive. Their life span is longer than adults: If a sixty year old patient has excessive radiation, by the time the injury reveals itself in twenty years, that patient may have died from other causes.

Diagnostic x-rays, especially fluoroscopic ones, used in people from infancy to age thirty, should be absolutely essential. X-ray treatments should likewise be used sparingly.

The disease Leukemia has been diagnosed in the children who survived the atom bombs in Japan in 1945. Likewise, Leukemia has been observed in American Children who were treated with x-rays. Cancer of the thyroid gland has been observed in children who were given x-ray treatment for tonsillitis, adenoids, thymus gland enlargement, etc. No benign condition should be treated by radiation. I can think of no excuse for exposing a child to radiation for a condition like enlarged tonsils or adenoids.

Of course, such treatments are very profitable. They present a very financially rewarding course for doctors to follow.

Skin conditions should not be treated with x-ray. Not in adults and not in children. Acne can be treated in safer ways than roentgen rays! Birthmarks on babies often disappear by the time the child reaches five. Other treatments are safer and effective. Ringworm can be treated by safer methods than radiation.

Children's bones are growing and are more susceptible to x-ray damage than adult's bones. X-rays have been used too, often by pediatricians, dermatologists, and dentists. "The younger the child, the greater is the sensitivity to radiation."[6]

Any doctor who uses radiation on children should discuss its hazard with the parents. Any doctor and any patient should ask themselves, "Is the possible end result of this treatment more hazardous to my health and life span than the condition for which it is being used?" If the answer is "Yes," radiation is not preventive medicine, it is a hazard.

A petroleum-derived protein called Torutein is used as a flavor enhancer or a food ingredient. This protein yeast culture is grown on hydrocarbons, which are distilled from crude oil. It is listed under present labeling laws as a flavor enhancer.

Sometimes it is called Torula yeast. It has never been proven free of toxic or carcinogenic effects. It is banned in Italy, Japan, and England. It is found in American food like La Choy Foods, French's Croutons, Prince's Macaroni, and Gerber Baby foods!

Lotions and shampoos contain Ethanolamines as wetting agents. It has been shown that these amines can nitroside to form a carcinogen called Nitrosodiethanolamine. Excess risk of cancer of the lung and bladder can result from constant use of such lotions and shampoos.

Beauticians are exposed to them in their work. Nitrosamine levels have been found in Johnson's Baby Lotion. It would be better for babies and small children if lotions used on them contained non-nitrogen Glycerol. Every possible way or reducing exposure to carcinogens on babies and small children should be pursued. All cosmetics used on children should be closely monitored. What is wrong with cornstarch like our grandmothers used?

Cancer in children should be a prime consideration when new products are introduced. The Consumer Product safety Commission was informed by a panel of independent scientists that the chemical DEHP (Di-2 Ethylhexyephalate) can cause cancer in rats.

It is potentially dangerous to humans. It is used in pacifiers, squeeze toys, and crib bumper pads, baby pants, covers, mattresses, and teething rings.

What did the Commission do with this information? Spokesman Lou Brott did not commit to any action from the agency. This, in spite of the fact that the panel said, "As DEHP is an animal carcinogen, it must be potentially carcinogenic to humans."

Studies have shown that 137 million products for children were distributed and they contained between 5.3 million and 12.9 million pounds of DEHP. Why the delay in banning it? There should be no delay. No consideration should be given to industry when the issue is cancer in children– or adults!

Dr. Langley Spurlock, Director of Biomedical and Environmental programs for the Chemical Manufacturer's Association, said he would give a child a pacifier containing DEHP and not worry about it at all.

He agreed it causes cancer in high doses in rats. But denied that it is a carcinogen for humans. The scientist's report said it resulted in liver cancer in mice and rats. Epidemiological studies have not addressed its human carcinogenity.

They should have. I think these people should visit a hospital's cancer ward for children. I wonder why the Consumer Product Safety Commission would pay more attention to an industry's spokesman than to scientists? The issue is the life and death of the innocents: OUR CHILDREN.

CHAPTER SIX

The Fda Is A Fraud

It would be the understatement of the year to say that the Food and Drug Administration has failed American consumers. This agency has withheld information. It has deceived and betrayed the people for whom it was founded to help.

The FDA has never enforced the Delaney clause of the Federal Food, Drug, and Cosmetic Art. This failure has been to the detriment of the health and life span of American citizens.

The Delaney Amendment became law in 1958. It states: "No additive shall be deemed safe if it is found to induce cancer when ingested by man or animal, or if it is found, after tests which are appropriate for the evaluation of the safety of food additives, to induce cancer in man or animal."

Today our food, drugs, and cosmetics are laced with carcinogens. We are all guinea pigs.

A specific example of the attitude of the FDA is the way DES (diethylstilbestrol) was handled. DES is a synthetic hormone and a powerful carcinogen. When pellet implants of DES were banned in 1973, the DES manufacturers obtained a court order reversing the ban.

The FDA did not contest the ban. When failure for this betrayal of consumers, the FDA commissioner, Herbert L. Ley made the arrogant remark, "I am not going to tell you the FDA has devised the perfect system for keeping chemicals out of our foods. You'll simply have to live with it."

Such betrayal helps explain why cancer is taking such a toll. We "simply are not living with carcinogens in our food." We sicken and we die from them.

The national Institute of Environmental Health Sciences has

37

recommended that mutagenic testing of food additives and pesticides are made mandatory. Dr. W.C. Hueper of the National Cancer Institute stated emphatically, "No one can establish a dose for carcinogens so small that it is safe."

We have no protection from dangerous food additives as long as the FDA insists on a demonstration of the harm an additive can cause before removing it from the GRAS (Generally Regarded as Safe) list.

It would be a more rational policy to demand that an additive be proven safe *before* placing it on the GRAS list. The present backward way of doing things is in effect malfeasance and nonfeasance of duty on the part of the FDA employees who are paid to protect the consumer.

The GRAS list is meaningless. GRAS should stand for "Generally Risky and Suicidal". This list should not be a determining factor for allowing additives in our food.

What kind of finagling and lobbying goes on? Why such indifference to the health of the citizens? Food manufacturers do not go through a long program of filing a petition with the FDA to clear their product for acceptance on this list. As a matter of fact, some manufacturers help the FDA evaluate their products. The Flavor and Extract manufacturing Association helps evaluate its own products. This is conflict of interest. The fox guards the hen house.

One of the lame alibis given is that the doses are so small that they are safe. There is no safe dose of poison. Another alibi is the theory that chemicals, which hurt laboratory animals, will not hurt men. This was proven wrong with many chemicals like arsenic and chromate to name two.

The standard alibi of food manufacturers and FDA executives is "the product was tested on laboratory animals and this does not prove it dangerous to mankind." Such an assumption is not realistic. For example, thalidomide damaged many unborn human babies in Europe. Efforts to railroad it through to public use by doctors in America were blocked by Dr. Frances Kelset. Women are ten times more sensitive to Thalidomide than mice. This was proven in tests on pregnant mice.

Spokesmen for the National Institute in Bethesda, Maryland now believe that forty to sixty percent of all human cancers are now thought to be diet-related. This is horrifying because the use of chemical additives has increased fifty percent. Americans eat more chemicalized food than any people in the world.

Since our government will not protect us, we should resolve to protect ourselves. The best cure for sickness is prevention. Knowledge is our best weapon. An English doctor told me, "You Americans eat your cancer." We can change this situation. We can do our homework. We can learn to identify dangerous additives. This will not be easy.

There are almost six thousand additives in our food. The FDA rules are not even logical. Some additives must be on labels, others do not require labeling. The public has no access to FDA files about studies on the toxic properties of additives. Still, we can consult the works of writers who have done independent research. We should protest to our representatives the fact that the scientific data on additives between industry and the United States Department of Agriculture is not in the public domain.

I would like to deal with some of the instances, which show a ruthless disregard for the public welfare. An additive, which has been proven dangerous, is ever present in our food, and its use is increasing. This additive is called Carrageenan. It is listed in salad dressing, cheese, sherbert, and ice cream. It is used in Vinegar, wine, and beer to control foam. This has been tested on laboratory animals and induced fatal ulcerative colitis. When fed to guinea pigs, it caused collagen granuloma. It is in infant formula powder. Why?

Let's examine DEP– Diethyl Pyrocarbonate. This additive is tasteless. It is used in beer, wine, and malt liquor. It is a co-carcinogen. When combined with other compounds it becomes carcinogenic. It reacts with ammonia to form urethan, an established carcinogen. Once urethan is formed in food, it stays there. It can break down and form intermediate products, one of which is dyethyl carbonate. When this was injected into hamsters, it showed teratogenicity.

DEP was banned in Sweden in 1971 because research conduced damaging evidence regarding BVO.

When it was fed into the diet of rats at a level of 0.59, it interfered with their metabolism. It produced high fat deposits in their kidneys and hearts. When fed to pigs, it was stored in their spleens with high concentrates in the pancreas, lungs, liver, and heart.

Studies made by the Canadian Food and Drug Directorate showed adverse changes in rats given low levels of BVO. For eighty days they suffered growth retardation, anemia, enlargement of the heart, kidney and spleen. Animals given BVO at a 2.5 feeding level showed arrested testicular development.

In January of 1970, the Canadian Minister of Health ordered reduction of its use. In February of 1970, British officials removed BVO from the list of permitted stabilizers and in September of that year announced it would no longer be permitted in food and drink.

In the wake of these findings what happened in the United States of America? In 1970 Charles Edwards, the Food and Drug Administration Commissioner said, "The Canadian and British studies were inconclusive." He allowed American food and beverage processors to continue using BVO pending further study.

Senator Abraham Ribicoff said, "The American people have generally assumed that new food additives have been tested by the government and licensed as safe. This proves to be anything but the case."

Dr. Samuel S. Epstein of the Children's Cancer Research Foundation and the Harvard Medical School believes consumer protection laws should involve testing the safety of food additives BEFORE allowing them to be used. The present system uses the consumers as test animals, putting the profit of the food seller first, public safety second.

An example of this was the way that cyclamates were removed from beverages years after it was proven they caused liver cancer in laboratory animals. Dr. Jacqueline Verret, the biochemist whose testimony had them banned, laid her job on the line when she spoke out. Her book *Eating May be Dangerous to Your Health* was quickly suppressed. Oil of Calamus, a carcinogen, was not banned until long after its carcinogenicity was established. Lithium Chloride was banned only after fatalities were linked to it. NDGA (Nordinhydroguaidretic Acid) caused severe kidney damage. It was removed from the GRAS list long after this was proven. Saffrole, which caused liver cancer, was removed after people died.

What happened with MSG– Monosodium Glutamate? Both the Gerber and Heinz companies were adding MSG to baby food. Dr. Jean Mayer denounced the use of MSG in baby food.

Herbert Ley, the FDA Commissioner tried to justify its usage. He was challenged by Ralph Nader's research group. Jim Turner, head of this group, said, "Clearly MSG should not be in baby food– and should have been removed as soon as doubts were raised about its safety."

MSG was removed from baby food in October, 1969, five months after reports were made that it caused brain damage in laboratory mice. It was removed only because of public pressure after Nader's group testified before a Senate hearing on its danger. It was not removed because the FDA was conscientiously doing its job. It was removed because Ralph Nader's Center for Study of Responsive Law investigated the FDA and testified about its negligence.

The FDA has a long history of negligence. I could go on with a list of sins it has committed against consumers. The dreary tale of FDA's betrayal of American consumers is an ongoing story. Examine the situation today with artificial food colors.

The biggest failures of the FDA so far? The failure to remove all artificial colors and sodium nitrites from the food supply.

In 1907 the Federal Food and Drugs Act began to study whether or not to certify coal tars used in food colors. Coal tar is carcinogenic.

In 1938, the need for color certification was written into law. In 1960, the color amendments called for the retesting of all food colors.

Prior to 1981, the FDA was the sole agency with the power to enforce laws relating to food, drugs and cosmetics. Then Ronald Reagan gave power to the Secretary of Health and Human Services to approve or reject FDA regulations. In so doing, the Reagan administration illegally undermined the FDA's ability to protect the health and safety of the American public.

Recently, a House committee accused the Reagan administration of illegally allowing the continued use of six known cancer-causing dyes in food, drugs, and cosmetics. They are red dye numbers 3, 8, 9, 19, 37, and orange dye number 17.

The FDA reported findings that these six additives cause cancer in laboratory animals. Representative Ted Weiss (D., NY) said, "This report reflects Congress' bipartisan view that health and human services has blatantly violated Federal Law in failing to ban six potentially hazardous dyes."

Margaret Heckler, Secretary of H.H.S. under the Reagan administration, offered no explanation why the dyes have not been banned. The most infamous of the dyes, red dye number 3 is used in maraschino cherries.

The maraschino cherry producers, as well as the drug and cosmetics industries lobbied to keep the dangerous dyes in use.

Industry pressure caused H.H.S. to reverse the FDA recommendations that the dyes be banned.

The House committee said continued use of the dyes violates the twenty-five year old laws that prohibit the use of color additives found to cause cancer in laboratory animals.

These laws require manufacturers to prove with reasonable certainty that the additives are safe. Industry claims about the safety of these additives are unsubstantiated.

The House said that additional review is "patently unnecessary and will in effect subvert if not completely paralyze enforcement of the nation's public health and safety laws."

Years ago, it was learned that sodium nitrite is a powerful carcinogen. It combines with amines in the body to create nitrosamines, which are very heavily carcinogenic. Read labels and what do you see? Sodium nitrite. It is heavily used in meats like hot dogs, sausage, salami, and bologna.

It is time to abolish the GRAS list and start over. We have in our food supply today, chemical additives capable of causing the following disastrous effects: Kidney damage, elevation of blood pressure, cardiac disturbances, reduction of fertility and virility, ulcerative colitis, and damage to the central nervous system. This is a partial list.

Many of these chemicals are banned in Canada, banned in Spain, banned in England, banned in France, banned in Russia, and so on.

The FDA has some insidious practices. Their policies are mysterious, indeed. There is a policy of "Provisional Listing." While years of scientific investigation drag by, artificial colors are used under this policy.

The tactic of reclassification was tired. When Dr. Jacqueline Verrett wanted cyclamates banned, the FDA tried to reclassify them as drugs. Congressman L.H. Fountain insisted they be classified as foods and they were banned.

There is a dodge called "The Interim Food Additive Order." Additives found harmful are removed from the GRAS list and put on this interim list, so testing can go on and on while the additives are used. This standard procedure is a violation of the law.

The FDA "Guidelines for Safety" state that there are safety margins. These safety margins are a myth. They are not determined by scientific data. We need a new agency to protect public safety.

The history of the FDA is a long record of dismal failure. There

42

has been no commitment to enforcement of laws already on the books. These are laws, which were passed to protect the American people. There has been betrayal of the people as evidenced in cases I described. The betrayal continues.

The FDA has a new commissioner, Dr. David Kessler. He spoke at a convention in the summer of 1991 in Palm Beach, Florida. He said, "I am here today to tell you that I place a high priority on enforcing the law. Today, the U.S. Attorney's office in Minneapolis, Minnesota is filing on FDA's behalf a seizure action against Proctor and Gamble's Citrus Hill Fresh Choice Orange Juice. The use of the term 'fresh' is false and misleading."

Dr. Kessler's friend, an attorney named Stuart Pape said, "Going after large companies and being tough have been part of a well considered strategy to increase the credibility and morale of the agency."

Tough? The freshness of orange juice or any juice is important for people who are allergic to chemicals used to make connections. But this problem is a tremendous trifle in the face of the fact that known carcinogens have been, and still are allowed in our food legally.

It might have been more in the public interest if Dr. Kessler's first announcement had been that the agency would make seizures of food containing known carcinogens. I would be more assured that he is the right person to be entrusted with the health of American consumers. Why did he fail to ban dangerous pesticides that pollute our fruits and vegetables? What is his policy on additives that are known mutagens and teratogens? Why has he failed to ban them? Why has he allowed irradiation of foods?

The White House and Congress act pleased with Dr. Kessler's performance. I am not convinced that anything about his performance is conducive to lowering cancer rates.

In fairness to Dr. Kessler, the FDA is grossly under-staffed and under-funded. It should be granted the funds it needs to become effective. Better yet, it should be abolished and funds allocated to an agency which will be independent of agribusiness and the pharmaceutical companies. Funds and staff should be given to a new agency.

Dr. Kessler's priorities are superficial. He needs more than money and a larger staff. He needs to face urgent priorities. It is

43

interesting to note that Dr. Kessler is concerned with labeling. He wants truth in labeling. He wants the labels on products to mean what they say. He wants fiber content listed. He wants the number of calories derived from fat listed. He wants consumers protected from misleading labels.

There are many such labels today. Some packages that say "natural" have only one natural ingredient and several artificial ones. Some labels claim "no preservatives," then list Xanthan gum or artificial colors. It is good that Dr. Kessler wants to increase consumer awareness of a healthier diet, but this will mean truth in labeling must be enforced in order to succeed.

There are some foods for which it is impossible to label. How do you label a bunch of fresh grapes? The pesticides on grapes are a powerful cancer threat. The towns of McFarland, Fowler and Earlimart, California are located in the heart of California's table grape growing region. Cancer causing pesticides in this area has increased cancer in children. Diagnosed cancer in Earlimart, a town of 4,000 people, is 1,200% above the expected rate. [1] These pesticides lave a residue on grapes. More pesticides are sprayed on table grapes than any other crop. In 1988, twelve million pounds of pesticides were used on US grapes. [2]

Some of the pesticides sprayed on grapes are: Captan, Parathion, Phosdrin, Dinoseb, Methyl Bromide, Cyclodiene, Triazine, Aldicarb, and Carbofunans. These dangerous chemicals have no place in our food supply. They should be banned. The ban must be enforced.

Poisons like Orthene and Aldicarb are used on watermelons—even though they have been banned by law. Enforcement of pesticide use for workers and consumers is weak and often non-existent. A report in 1987 from the General Accounting Office (GAO) concludes that the government does not test for many of the pesticides currently being applied to the food we consume. It does not penalize growers who violate the law. I am personally boycotting grapes. Why should I have to avoid a health giving fruit because of corruption in our governmental agencies? Why has the FDA ignored the contamination of grapes with cancer-causing chemicals for so many years?

The U.S. Food and Drug Administration has failed to give the facts about food irradiation to the American people. This agency has withheld information from us. The fact is: Evidence has been shown that irradiation may promote the formation of a powerful carcinogen

44

called Aflatoxin.

Aflatoxin grows in vegetable spores and grains in humid climates. Studies in India revealed that Aflatoxin production was increased in stored wheat that had been irradiated. Aflatoxin causes cancer of the liver. According to the Environmental Protection Agency, Aflatoxin is 1,000 times more potent a carcinogen than EDB (Ethylene Di-Bromide) which the FDA banned.

How did the FDA claim food irradiation is safe? This agency reviewed more than 400 studies then decided to review only 69 of them. Thirty-two showed adverse effects, thirty-seven showed no damage. The FDA dismissed the studies showing adverse effects— then they dismissed thirty-two of the studies suggesting safety. On the use of the remaining five studies, the FDA pronounced irradiation safe.

Dr. John Gofman, Professor Emeritus of Medical Physics at the University of California, Berkeley, is a world-acknowledged authority on low-level radiation. He believes research to prove safety of irradiated food has never been done.

States Dr. Gofman, "the kind of epidemiological study required to find out whether or not a diet of irradiated food will increase (or decrease) the frequency of cancer or genetic injuries among humans simply has not been done. What is more, such a study is unlikely to be done because it would require controlling the diets of at least 200,000 humans of various age groups for at least thirty years and following their health histories for at least 50 years (preferably their full lifespans)".

We are all guinea pigs. Until such studies are done with humans.

The United States Army has researched irradiated foods. The FDA rejected the Army's research on irradiated pork back in 1968. Then they asked a company named Industrial BioTest to do research for them. By 1983, officials at I.B.T. were convicted of performing fraudulent research and suppression of unfavorable findings.

I.B.T. had conducted studies on irradiated strawberries, apples, pears, and papaya. These tests are used by the FDA to claim safety for irradiated foods— tests done by a firm that cheats!

A study done by Ral Tech, a branch of Ralston Purina in 1983 showed that mice who had been fed irradiated chicken had a tendency to get cancer of the testicles.

Despite this, the FDA has approved dosages of 300,000 RAD for spices, and 100,000 RAD for fruits and vegetables.

The excuse for this morally outrageous performance on the part of the FDA is "irradiation will reduce salmonella". The fact is that proper hygiene in producing and processing food will diminish salmonella. So will adequate cooking– no one has claimed that irradiation of food would be a way to reduce world hunger!

Little or no mention is made of the fact that the irradiation plants would pollute the air or contaminate the environment. How much study has been done on the risk of cancer from irradiation? Why has the Energy Department failed to release information to the public? Could it be due to the fact that the Energy Department will supply Cesium 137– which is a waste byproduct of nuclear reactors?

Has the FDA honestly conducted studies about the "safety" of irradiated food? Only five animal studies were conducted according to 1980 toxicological standards and these studies were flawed. The studies do not prove safety. Furthermore, they were done at lower doses than the FDA approved dose of 100,000 RAD. They are frauds. What these studies did reveal is that irradiated food has reduced levels of Vitamin E. The trust is– it is impossible to study the effect of irradiation on food in anything less twenty years of usage by thousands of humans.

Irradiation of foods causes the loss of Vitamins A, C, E, and B complex. When irradiated foods are cooked, there is more vitamin loss. We do not know what would happen if irradiated food was frozen. Any one eating irradiated foods should take vitamin supplements. More information on the nutritional "value" of irradiated food will become available as it is consumed.

Another consideration is the impact on the environment from plants where food is irradiated. Is it safe to work with radioactive isotopes? Will the safety regulations be enforced? What if there is a leak? How safely can Cobalt 60 and Cesium 137 be shipped to the plants?

Is there a threat of cancer? Already tests on laboratory mice have shown that malignant tumors can result from a steady diet of food that was nuked by Cesium 137. The health of the public has not been considered.

Irradiation has been advocated by the Department of Energy– D.O.E. Why? Certainly not to stop the growth of salmonella in our food. Has anyone heard of an epidemic of salmonella? There are tried

46

and true ways of preventing salmonella.

The D.O.E. has sly and disgusting motives for advocating irradiation. This agency wants to instigate a demand for Cesium 137– which is a byproduct of Plutonium extraction. Cesium 137 is used (as is Cobalt 60) as a source of gamma rays in food irradiation plants.

In 1982, congress banned the reprocessing of nuclear wastes as commercial wastes. The D.O.E. wants congress to allow the reprocessing of spent fuel to "help industry"– such as irradiation plants. The need for Cesium 137 will escalate so demand exceeds supply and congress will allow the D.O.E. to bypass the ban.

Over protests from doctors and scientists, the FDA –with encouragement from the Reagan Administration– approved irradiation of certain foods *AND DRUGS*! Plants had been using Cobalt 60. The D.O.E. started to use Cesium 137 as their gamma ray source in the food irradiation plants they were developing.

The Cesium 137 was part of a stockpile from military reactors. Wastes at the D.O.E. Hanford Nuclear Reservation near Richland, Washington and at a military reactor in Aiken, South Carolina. $5,000,000 was allowed for pilot projects (1987) and 1.7 million Curies of Cesium 137 was set aside for irradiation projects. The D.O.E. has much to gain from the irradiation of our food with *NUCLEAR GARBAGE.*

Food Irradiation is a cover up for weapons production! Weapons production creates the byproduct Cesium 137 and if food irradiation is legalized, there will be a shortage of Cesium 137 unless weapons production is increased!

In 1983, the House Armed Services Subcommittee issued a plan for utilizing nuclear byproducts. It stated "The measure of success (in the program) will be the degree to which this technology is implemented industrially and the subsequent demand created for Cesium 137."

This statement insinuates that the D.O.E. will deliver Cesium 137 even if it means violating the congressional ban on reprocessing nuclear wastes.

Military reactors generate a huge volume of radioactive waste. The disposal of this waste is one of the reasons the D.O.E. wants to irradiate our food with Cesium 137. It could save $1 billion on storage of such waste if it sells the Cesium 137 to a private plant that irradiates food.

General Foods, Beatrice– Hunt Wesson, and about thirty-two other companies have formed "the coalition for food irradiation." If they succeed in their efforts to hoodwink the consumers that nuclear food is safe, the D.O.E. will supply the Cesium 137.

Again, I want to stress that only Congress can stop the vicious sly plans to process nuclear waste from weapons material so it can be used to irradiate our food. Write your congressman to place a legal ban on irradiation.

Irradiation is banned in England. It is banned or severely restricted in Sweden, Germany, Denmark, and Australia. We must notify our congressman and senators that we want it banned here.

The latest insult to the American citizens from this corrupt agency is a new proposal for government regulations, which are oppressive. These regulations would allow the FDA to make wholesale seizures of substances not on the GRAS (generally regarded as safe) list. They would also allow seizures of substances for which a health claim is made.

These seizure procedures will begin in May 19993. The FDA wants state governments to be empowered to enforce these regulations. Officials in Texas are already raiding health food stores. This is gross hypocrisy because the GRAS list is fraudulent, composed of substances never proven safe.

How does the FDA presume to act this way? It is exceeding the mandate of Congress, which, in 1991, passed the Nutrition Labeling and Education Act. This will be referred to as the NLEA.

There are hidden problems in the NLEA. The first one is the replacement of the RDA (recommended daily allowance) with the RDI (reference daily intake). The food industry wants the RDI because it will lower the amount of vitamins and minerals added to food. This could result in nutritional deficiencies for the citizens.

Another problem is the desire of the FDA to dictate nutritional information. It wants to prevent such facts from use as the fact that prune juice is useful for irregularity or that fiber is useful to reduce the risk of getting heart disease or some cancers. In other words, the FDA wants to continue its practice of withholding information.

This tyrannical agency wants to use the NLEA to seize dietary supplements. The FDA wants to destroy the health food industry.

The power grab of the FDA is a violation of our rights. The

agency wants HR 3642 to be enacted. A Senate version of this is called HR 2135. These bills would allow the FDA to impose huge fines on doctors, retail stores, and manufacturers for violations of NLEA. These bills would allow the FDA to violate our constitutional rights to due process.

1. "The Cancer Industry– Unraveling the Politics", Ralph W. Moss, Paragon House, 1989
2. "Physicans' Desk Reference", Medical Economics Data Company, Inc., Montvale, NJ 07645
3. "The Cancer Industry– Unraveling the Politics", Ralph W. Moss, Paragon House , 1989, p. 85
4. "Cancer and Vitamin C," Ewan Cameron and Linus Pauling, W.W. Norton and Co., New York, 1979 p. 78
5. "Supernutrition," Richard Passwater, the Dial Press, New York, NY, 1975
6. "Cancer and Vitamin C," Ewan Cameron and Linus Pauling, W.W. Norton and Co., New York, 1979 p. 141

CHAPTER SEVEN

Silent Killers

We can become knowledgeable about food. We can boycott food products laced with carcinogenic preservatives and additives. We can refuse to use municipal water and buy bottled water. We can study drugs and demand that our doctors prescribe wisely.

We cannot stop breathing. We are at the "mercy" of the polluters who poison our air. We are at the "mercy" of the government regulatory agencies, which are supposed to enforce laws, which prohibit air pollution.

We can change this situation. We can monitor chemical plants and toxic waste landfills. We can demand the enforcement of the Federal Clean Air Act. The problem starts at the top. If the president of the United States wants the Clean Air Act enforced, he will appoint an honest administrator to head the Environmental Protection Agency. During the Reagan-Bush years, the EPA was run by lawless individuals who put the chemical industry's profits ahead of the public welfare.

Our air is infused with sulfides, hydrocarbons, and filth. Chlorofurocarbons, concoctions of soot, pesticides, gases, aerosols have even changed the color of the air. Toxic chemicals have created a brown haze over some citizens.

The result: millions of citizens live at highest risk of lung cancer and skin cancer. Millions of citizens have damaged immune systems. Technology was supposed to help the human race. Instead, it kills. A bird does not befoul its nest. Mankind must stop befouling the air—or perish.

Where are scientists who created these pollutants? Are they trying to undo the damage? Do they even acknowledge the problem?

The fact is: they are mainly silent. The protests over air pollution are coming from citizens who may not have scientific genius, but have enough common sense to know that **we must clean up the air.**

Section 112 of the Clean Air Act requires the EPA to protect the citizens from dangerous pollutants. This agency is a sham.

Dioxin levels in the soil near Midland, Michigan were six times higher than levels in the soil of Vietnam. The EPA declared they were "Not an acceptable risk". Dioxin is invisible. It is deadly. It is a silent killer. And it travels. Air moves. The Jet Stream can move at more than 100 miles an hour.

The polluting particles in the air do not stay near the chemical plants that discharge them. Wind usually flows eastward. Pollutants from a factory in Ohio or Michigan may move to New York or New Jersey or points east. There is no safety zone. And that is a tragedy.

The fact that the bureaucrats do not acknowledge the problem of air pollution is tragic. The fact that the bureaucrats do not enforce the law regulating industrialists who let the citizens sicken and die is tragic. The body count grows. That is more than a tragedy. It is moral outrage!

The United States of America is considered the wealthiest nation in the world. Sometimes, other nations speak enviously or our wealth. Unfortunately, some of our nation's wealth has been at the expense of the health and life spans of the citizens.

The technology that has brought prosperity is out of control. This technology has released poisonous chlorofuorocarbons into the air. This technology has damaged the ozone shield. This technology has caused environmental damage with resuctant environmental illnesses and death.

Skin cancer and other cancers have increased. The incidence of cancer has increased. Economic growth that increases the incidence of cancer is not acceptable.

We live at highest risk of getting cancer. In addition to poisoned food, drugs, and cosmetics, we breathe poisoned air. Air pollution as a cause of cancer has not been given adequate attention. This deadly problem has not been given regulation.

Federal laws about air pollution have not addressed the problem. Of the thousands of toxic chemicals, which pollute our air, only six have been given attention. They are: "Carbon monoxide, sulphur dioxide, and lead. [1]

51

The two largest chemical producers are DuPont and Dow Chemical Company. Dow is famous (infamous would be a better word) for developing the process that created Phenol. This chemical has by-products like orthophenylphenol and paraphenylphenol. [2]

Then Dow combined phenol with chlorine to form products called Chlorophenols. These are used in weed killers and products for prevention of mold and fungus.

The next deadly development was trichlorophenol. This is used in herbicides like 2,4,D and 2,4,5T. In the Vietnam War, this product was used and named "Agent Orange". Protests about these new chemical agents were first made by veterans of the Vietnam War. They claimed these chemicals caused cancer and birth defects.

The next silent killer from Dow— "We do great things for you" — Chemical Company was a compound, which formed during the manufacture of trichlorophenol. Called 2378TCDD, it is known as dioxide. This is the most toxic synthetic chemical known to man. [3] Dioxin caused the disaster at Love Canal.

TCDD— dioxin —has been studied and researched in laboratories by the Environmental Protection Agency. The EPA found that it was more toxic than cyanide. Animal studies proved that dioxin can have adverse effects on any organ in the body.

It is a carcinogen of such potency that it is without precedent. Dr. Barry H. Rumack, Director of the Rocky Mountain Poison Center in Denver, Colorado, said, "Dioxin is probably one of the most toxic chemicals known in the world." [4] Other authorities consider it the most toxic.

It is to the benefit of the human race that dioxin has been exposed as a killer. But why was this chemical compound used without being submitted to and researched by the EPA? Why was it exposed only after so much damage was done?

This compound causes degeneration of the thymus gland. It alters the mechanism that regulates food intake so that animals exposed to it eat too little and waste away.

In addition to being carcinogenic, dioxin is teratogenic (birth defect-causing). In Seveso, Italy, dioxin was accidentally released in 1976. [5] The people exposed to it developed chloracne and had spontaneous abortions. Birth defects like spina bifida and polydactyly (too many toes and fingers) were common.

In 1983, Dow stopped the manufacturing of the Herbicide 2,4,5,T which had released dioxin into the environment. This was **ten years after the EPA tried to regulate it.**

Dioxin is still in the soil and water. People have been indirectly exposed to it from eating animals and fish that ingested it.

Past exposures have left people with a body burden. Humans concentrate dioxin in their fat. The average body burden of dioxin if 5 to 10 PBT, and there is a strong possibility this is presenting an increased risk of cancer.

Dumping waste in the ground poisons both surface and ground water supplies. More commercials, industrial, and municipal waste will be burned. This increases dioxin production.

The waste burning facilities are called "resource recovery plants". These incinerators must maintain temperatures of 1600 F to keep dioxin in a range that will cause fewer than the "acceptable" estimate of six cancers per million people.

Citizens in every city should monitor the waste burning practices of their local sanitation department. We cannot make dioxin now present in the environment disappear. We can, however, insist that production of more dioxin be halted.

Another silent deadly killer is radon– a radioactive gas that occurs naturally. [6] Capable of building up to dangerous levels in houses, it causes thousands of deaths every year. These are avoidable deaths. To minimize the deadly effects of radon, changes in a house can be made. Such changes are not expensive. They are certainly less expensive than lung cancer.

Radon can seed into the house through the floor from the soil. It is a natural gas. It is not one of the man-made poisonous gases. Radon creates a hazard, which endangers houses, schools, and offices, all buildings in which people have to stay indoors a length of time.

When radon decays, it becomes polonium, which is an undesirable chemical element. Radon causes cancer. Studies of survivors of atomic bombing in Hiroshima and Nagasaki, Japan, prove this. Lung cancer and liver cancer are deadly. They are not as treatable as cancer in other organs. Sadly, radon is a common cause of cancer.

Radon can damage and break strands of DNA (Deoxyribo-Nucleic Acid). DNA controls the working and reproduction of cells. When DNA is damaged, the cells undergo mutations, which can lead to a pre-cancerous condition.

Cancer forms in stages. If cells are damaged by radiation and are

53

pre-cancerous, the introduction of any new carcinogen– say, "a chemical food additive– may cause the damaged, mutated cell to become cancerous. It is important to avoid Radon-caused mutations in the cells.

Radon itself does not stay in the lungs long. But when it decays to polonium, it can cause DNA damage in lung cells and lead to cancer.

The amount of radon coming from uranium mine tailings or radium painting is small. Most of it comes naturally from sail and rocks. The amount of radon coming to the surface is affected by moisture.

Occasionally indoor radon can come from tap water, natural gas, air, or even building materials. But this is not the way radon usually gets into houses.

Radon gets into a house because of the differences between air in the house and the air under the house. Wind and temperature can cause such air pressure differences. Any crack or hole in the floor admits radon. The type of rock and soild under a house determines radon levels– not the design of the house.

Radiation causes cancer in humans. Many studies have confirmed this. These studies were made with difficulty, because of the latency period.

In radon-caused lung cancer, the latency period averages twenty years.[7] No specific amount of radiation has been determined as needed to cause cancer. However, even at low dosage rates, radiation can cause cancer.

Sources of information on human lung cancer are the studies of survivors of Hiroshima and Nagasaki. There were also studies of coal miners. These confirmed that radon causes lung cancer. Smokers who are exposed to radon have an increased risk of lung cancer.

The way to reduce the risk of lung cancer is to reduce the level of radon in the house. There are radon detectors on the market. The charcoal canister radon detector and the Alpha-Track detector are inexpensive. The charcoal detectors are sold by Key Technology, PO Box 562, Jonestown, PA 17038 (Air detector - $19.99, Water detector- $19.99).

The Alpha –Track detector is sold by Terradex Corporation, 3 Science Rd., Glenwood, IL 60425. (Air detector and water detector $29.95).

When a reading has been made by the detector, a level above 4

Pci/s requires a second reading to be made. This follow up should be made by an Alpha Track detector. If the second reading confirms the first, changes should be made in the house.

To make a house safe from radon, the owner must locate the radon entry points. These could be cracks in the floor or holes where pipes are installed. When a house has a crawl space, floor cracks must be detected and sealed. Gaps between wall and floor sumps are radon entry points.

Radon can be monitored in a house by using a track etch detector. Companies sell detectors, which measure radon pollution. Teradex Corp., 460 North Wiget Lane, Walnut Creek, CA 94508 makes a radon monitoring system, as does the University of Pittsburg. This can be obtained through Radon Protection Service, Radon Project, Pittsburgh, PA 15260.

States have radon programs. Some states have information programs. Some have programs that are actively assisting homeowners with radon problems. For a list of the locations of each state's radon program, consult "Radon Risk and Remedy," by David J. Brenner, W.H. Freeman and Co., New York, NY.

If unacceptable levels of radon are detected, corrective steps must be taken. To prevent radon gas from filtering into the house, all cracks in basement walls and concrete slabs should be sealed with polymeric caulks.

Crawl spaces have to be ventilated. Solid wood should be used instead of plywood when building. Air cleaners on the market cost about $350.00. They are not usually adequate.

Subfloor suction involves inserting pipes through holes in a concrete slab basement floor. A fan at the end of the pipe outside of the house draws air away from the soil. Most houses require more than one pipe. The rule is one pipe for every 700 square feet of floor.

Radon can enter the water supply. Surface water is safer than underground water. Municipal water supplies use underground water which has low levels of radon.

Hot water releases more radon than cold water. The problem of radon in water usually is found in individual well water, or in small communities.

Most drinking water does not contain harmful levels of radon.

Nuclear power plants cause radiation, but not in the high doses that radon does. To decrease lung cancer, radon must be reduced in our houses.

Radon is one of many silent killers that invade our homes, schools, and office buildings. Aerosol products, formaldehyde, asbestos, sulfur dioxide, carbon monoxide are some of the pollutants that cause "sick building syndrome".

Indoor air pollution is as dangerous as outdoor air pollution. The National Academy of Sciences estimates that the air pollution in buildings adds a cost of $100 billion annually to the cost of health care. [8]

Outdoor air pollution is dangerous, but we spend 90 percent of our time indoors. So, we must pay attention to the odorless, colorless pollutants that are poisoning the air in our homes.

One source of indoor air pollution is the gas-burning appliance. Gas stoves and dryers release carbon dioxide and carbon monoxide into the air. Gas stoves with pilot lights release these poisons constantly.

A study by Frank Speizer of Harvard University was conducted with 8,000 children ages 6 to 10. This study linked impaired lung function with the presence of gas stoves.[9]

Kerosene space heaters release sulfur dioxide and nitrogen dioxide and should not be used.

Another silent killer that invades homes is formaldehyde. It can come from foam insulation, fiberwood, textiles, paper, tobacco smoke and especially plywood.

A sealant should be used on unfinished wood products like cabinets and stairs. Formaldehyde can enter the blood stream. It can irritate the eyes, nose, and throat.

It can cause asthma. In research laboratory work, it has been found to cause cancer of the nose in laboratory rats. The National Academy of Sciences decided that formaldehyde is a potential human carcinogen.[10]

Growing house plants is a good defense against indoor air pollution because plants absorb it.

Aerosol sprays in cans release hydrocarbons, which are toxic. The human race lived for centuries without aerosol sprays. They are an unnecessary danger and should be avoided.

Asbestos consists of silicate mineral fibers. It was used commonly until its dangers were discovered in the early 1960's. When asbestos fibers enter the lungs, they cause the disease asbestosis, and lung cancer can develop. An effort is being made to remove asbestos from public buildings like schools and post offices.

A physicist from the EPA, Lance Wallace, said, "The American home is more of a toxic waste dump than any area around a chemical plant."

There are other highly toxic pollutants found in the American home. Carbon monoxide comes from faulty furnaces, unvented gas stoves and exhaust fumes from attached garages.

To avoid poisoning from carbon monoxide, the furnace and chimney should be inspected and cleaned every year. Keep a window open an inch or two. Vent gas stoves to the outside, or run a kitchen fan. Do not run a car in the garage unnecessarily.

Methylene chloride is found in paint thinners and strippers. Such products must not be stored in a garage. If you do not have an outdoor shed, throw unused containers away.

Benzo-Pyrene comes from wood stoves and tobacco. To avoid it, smoke in well-ventilated rooms, and have wood stoves cleaned often. It is better not to smoke.

Paradichlorobenzene is used in mildew retardants, mothballs, and air fresheners. Avoid these products.

Chloroform is found in drinking water treated with chlorine. It is also found in disinfectants and household cleaners. It is best not to use city water for drinking. Houshold cleaners and disinfectants should be used in well-ventilated areas.

An under-the-sink charcoal water filter should be installed. Avoid taking long, hot showers and baths.

Tetrachloroethylene is in dry cleaning fluid. It is safer to air dry cleaned clothing outside before wearing them.

Nitrogen oxide comes from unvented gas stoves. Vent gas stoves to the outside or run a fan while cooking.

Trichloroethane is another poison in aerosol spray. Pump activated sprays are preferable.

Benzene comes from tobacco smoke and gasoline vapors. Smoke in well-ventilated rooms. Never warm up a car in an attached garage.

Lung cancer has a very poor cure rate. You can reduce the risk of lung cancer by reducing the levels of toxic fumes in your home.

Carbon tetrachloride is used in some shampoos, in dry cleaning and in anesthesia. It forms deadly phosgene gas, which can cause poisoning, and death. Study the label on hair shampoos.

One of the most vicious silent, tasteless, invisible and odorless killers is mercury. The fumes from mercury can kill. When mercury was used to make felt, it drove the hatters mad.

In 1953, mercury used in handling seafood killed Japanese fisherman. A chemical plant dumped mercury, which is 30 times heavier than water. It sank to the bottom of Minamata Bay and poisoned the fisherman.

Methyl Mercury is worse than organic mercury. It is deadly and builds up in tissues.

In sweden, methyl mercury seed dressings were used as fungicides. Birds died and people got sick from eating the meat of animals that had eaten contaminated crops.

In 1966, Sweden held an international conference on mercury. It was attended by five U.S. government scientists. Sweden acted and banned mercury-based fungicide.

The United States did not act. Our government agency studied mercury– and people died. Our governmental agencies study us to death.

Mercury damages brain cells and the central nervous system. The hazards of mercury do not lessen in time. They accumulate. Damage from mercury dumped into the river by industry is **not temporary.** The effects of mercury poisoning of fish will remain for years.

In 1989, mercury was found in the food chain of the Everglades in Florida. A panther died after eating contaminated fish. Signs were posted warning anglers not to eat fish taken from the area.

Man is poisoning his world. When the fauna in the Everglades are not safe, it is later than we think.

Mercury is used in the manufacture of electrical equipment. It is used in agricultural pesticides, disinfectants, mildew proofing, caustic soda, chlorine. The limit for mercury residues in food should be zero.

The Federal Drug Administration set a limit for mercury concentration at .5 parts per million. This is three times the limit set in Russia or allowed by the World Health Organization– W.H.O.

The most obiquitous silent killer is in the United States is nuclear waste. It is invisible, odorless, and everywhere. Radioactivity is measured by Curie. The Curie of our nuclear garbage is in the billions. There is enough to kill every living creature in the country. At the present rate of accumulation, there will soon be enough to kill everyone on the planet.

The nuclear industry has not found a way to dispose of its waste. No technology has been devised to isolate and dispose of this waste. It can cause cancer, birth defects, and other diseases. Our radioactive garbage endangers us all. However, the Atomic Energy Commission was unconcerned about the problem.

The National Academy of Sciences is an organization of engineers and scientists who study science issues for federal agencies. This group asserts the problem of nuclear waste has been solved.

The stark truth is: No technology has been developed for the safe disposal of nuclear waste.

Methods of disposal for deadly waste have been unsuccessful. Attempts to bury it in the land have resulted in contamination of the land. Trenches collapsed in a nuclear waste grave near Chicago, Illinois and after the disposal site was closed, tritium showed up in nearby wells.

Plutonium buried in Kentucky seeped off into streams and nearby property. This is a powerful poison, which scientists claimed was "immobile".

The fact that the mass production of nuclear waste had begun without technology to dispose of it, was now clear. Nuclear waste is put in trucks and driven around the country with no single governmental agency responsible for enforcing safety regulations.

Our government has been consistent about its betrayal of the people— in the problem of nuclear waste disposal. It has withheld information. It has lied. It has failed to enforce safety regulations. When radioactive liquid leaked out of underground storage tanks at Hanford, Washington, the lie was told that waste problems were manageable.

The Atomic Energy commission claimed, "In more than a decade of tank storage at Hanford, no leaks have been detected. The federal government has lied in an effort to hide failures and discredit any research reports that warn about the dangers of radioactive waste.

A study was made of 500,000 males who died between 1950 and 1971 in Washington. The staff physician for the Washington State Department of Social and health Services reached the conclusion that workers at Hanford had a greater chance to die of cancer than other males in the state.

Dr. Samuel Milham Jr. who made the study, was informed by the A.E.C. that it would be better not to publish his study. He did publish it in a short form. Others who predicted thousands of cases of cancer and leukemia per year were fired or suppressed.

Of all the silent killers released into the air we breathe, water we drink, food we eat, drugs we take, nothing is more pervasive than radiation.

It causes leukemia and most types of cancer. Strontium enters the bones. Radon and plutonium invades the lungs. Iodine reaches the tyroid glands. As stockpiles of radioactive waste accumulate, we are all at risk. Tragically, so are the unborn.

Genetic disease from radiation could include cancer, mental retardation, schizophrenia, dwarfism, and other maladies.

1.   "The Toxic Cloud, Michael H. Brown, Harper and Row, 10 East 53rd Street, New York, NY, 1987, p. 7.
2.   Ibid, p. 17.
3.   Ibid, p. 19.
4.   "Dioxin-Agent Orange", Michael Gough, Plenum Press, New York, NY, 1986, p. 14.
5.   "House Dangerous— Indoor Pollution in Your Home and Office," Ellen S. Greenfield, Vintage Book, New York, NY, 1987, p. 17.
6.   "Radon, Risk and Remedy," David S. Brenner, W.H. Freeman and Company, Preface.
7.   Ibid, p. 80.
8.   "House Dangerous— Indoor Pollution in Your Home and Office," Ellen S. Greenfield, Vintage Books, New York, NY, 1987, p. 4.
9.   Ibid, p. 17.
10. Ibid, p. 151.
11. "Forevermore Nuclear Waste In America," Donald L. Bartlette and James B. Steele, William Norton and Company, New York, NY, 1085, p. 66.
12. Ibid, p. 69.

CHAPTER EIGHT

Acid Rain

Sulphur dioxide interacts. It combines with moisture in the atmosphere to become sulphuric acid H2SO4. Oxides of nitrogen become HNO3 – nitric acid. As these acids fall and float among clouds and air currents, they are aerosols, waiting as acid in the sky.

Sulphuric acid and nitric acid are corrosive acids, invidious and invisible. They have altered the composition of rain and snow and fog. Now, we have acid rain, acid smog, and acid sleet. Dust can also become acidic.

This acid rain and moisture falls on water and turns it into a chemical mess. Fish and frogs perish. This acid moisture corrodes buildings. It falls on the earth and upsets the balance of the soil. Such acid moisture damages human lungs. Acid rain enters the soil and pollutes it.

In Germany in 1981, a conference was called. Scientists and government officials met to discuss a survey with the Minister of Food, Agriculture, and Forestry. The survey was made public in November, 1982. A report "Forest Damage Due to Air Pollution" stated that 7.7% of forest area had been damaged.

A second survey had worse results. It related that the damage had increased four times. In addition to usual causes of forest damage (Pests, weather, etc.), the survey reported a new cause of damage. "There are indications that atmosphere pollutants and their conversion products are a major cause of forest damage. Sulphur dioxide is probably the most important.

Not only does acid rain damage leaves and bark, it gets into the soil and damages the roots of trees. The roots are not able to let moisture flow to the trunks and leaves of the trees. Acid rain is a silent killer of our forests.

Acid rain kills people. Two percent of the deaths per year in the United States and Canada might be attributed to atmospheric sulphur particulate pollution. Thousands suffer from lung disease because of this pollution.

Pre-existing asthma is aggravated as is bronchitis and heart disease when sulphate pollutes the air.

The price of pollution control is not as high as the electric companies, chemical plants and others want us to believe.

In 1979, the EPA's Douglas Costle said, "Pollution control could have cost the electric utilities to increase the average residential electric bill $1.20 a month.

Acid rain abatement methods are primarily: 1) Coal washing and 2) Fuel switching. Coal washing involves pulverizing coal to be burned. It is passed through mesh screens and wetted down. This allows sulphur-bearing pyrites to sift out from lighter coal. This reduces sulphur emissions.

Fuel switching is more effective and economical than installing scrubbers and coal washing. But switching to western coal might cause an economic depression in Ohio, West Virginia and Pennsylvania. So it is not widely used.

Other newer technologies for emission reduction are being developed. Chemical coal cleaning, coal liquefaction and gasification, ocean-thermal conversion and fluidized bed combustion have been used.

Co-generation is an industrial system that produces heat, energy, and electricity from the same fuel source. This doubles the usefulness of the fuel.

How has the government acted to protect the citizens? It has done very little. In fact, some government agencies have lied about the dangers. A member of the Atomic Energy Committee, William F. Libby, said, "People have got to learn to live with the facts of life and part of the facts of life are fallout."

The same A.E.C. refused to believe that radioactive fallout killed the sheep in Utah in 1955. Documents proving the sheep were killed by fallout were hidden. Evidence was suppressed. A cover-up was attempted.

The Atomic Energy Commission behaves as despicably when men, women, and children die from radioactive exposure. This agency tried to cover up the tragedy when workers at Hanford, Washington died of cancer and leukemia.

Government agencies do not care about the safety and lives of the citizens. They have been bought and paid for by private industry.

These agencies will not police the atomic power industry. They do not admit to leaks in radioactive waste storage facilities. When tragedies happen, they juggle the statistics.

The National Academy of Sciences does not concede that radiation is a threat. The Environmental Protection Agency is convinced storage units are safe. The Department of Energy wants to irradiate our food. The Nuclear Regulatory Committee downgrades hazards.

The people who staff these agencies are committing malfeasance and nonfeasance in office and cancer increases.

These agencies should be abolished. New agencies should be formed – and scrutinized by citizens' advisory boards.

New agencies should be held accountable for their decisions. The people working in these agencies should listen and respond to citizens' concerns and protests.

Our present government agencies serve special interests. This deadly situation is intolerable. If no change is made, the silent killers will continue to kill.

CHAPTER NINE

Water, Water Everywhere But Not A Drop To Drink

Water, water, everywhere, but not a drop to drink. This is the situation today. No life survives without water. Now our water is so polluted it kills the fish and is not safe to swim in, let alone, to drink.

One-fifth of the world's fresh water lies in the Great Lakes. These lakes are called the "The Fifth Coast." How has the human race treated these important bodies, which are really seas, not lakes?

Lake Erie almost died. It was a sewer so vile that it was a fire hazard. Logs, tires, paints and chemicals were dumped into it. Detergent foam reached eight feet high. It was a sewer of sludge.

Lake Erie is older than the other Great Lakes. Its bed does not reach below sea level. It is only two-hundred and ten feet deep. The watershed is on earth, not rock.

The water tasted like rotting vegetation. The major tributaries are polluted. Pollutants do not always run to streams, rivers, lakes through pipes. They can run off over the ground and through the ground. Rain can stir them up and pour them on the ground.

Only Lake Superior escaped major problems. Detroit's sewer system was bad. So were the systems in Toledo, Cleveland and Buffalo. But the problems they caused Lake Superior were not as severe as other lakes.

Lake Michigan became polluted with Ammonium Bisulfite from paper mills. A small auto parts plant was discharging TCE into drinking water wells from 1973 – 1978.

TCE is a strong carcinogen which can cause heart and kidney disease, as well as cancer. The cost of closing the wells, $140,000.00, was not borne by the auto parts plant. The city with help from the federal government, paid for it.

The taxpayers were poisoned by ruthless businessmen, then had to pay to undo the damage that they had caused. TCE is a strong poison, so the citizens had to pay to have it cleaned up. It is Trichloroethylene.

Toxaphene, a strong pesticide, pollutes Lakes Superior, Michigan and Huron. It shows in the fish. Our lakes are polluted by ammonia, phenol, lead, cyanide, chronium, to name a few of the poisonous chemicals we drink.

The Dow Chemical Company in Midland, Michigan, dumps dioxins and PCB's into the tributaries of Lake Huron. Lake Ontario is polluted with drainage from the Love Canal and other dumps.

Lake Ontario was also polluted by Mirex. This is one of the most dangerous chemicals ever developed. It causes cancer and is tetragenic, (can cause birth defects). It is a pesticide used to kill fire ants. It poisoned the fish, as well as the water.

The Pesticide Industry is a multi-billion dollar a year business. Insecticides, fungicides, rodenticides are used promiscuously. When absorbed by water and carried to the bottom, they are like malignancies.

Water moves. Currents move. Eddies swirl. There is continuous movement of water. Water can pick up chemicals and can carry them. When it holds them we call the process absorption.

The sad fact about the pollution of our water is that the use of such poisons is not necessary. History tells us that before chemical pesticides were developed, farmers used safe methods to protect their crops.

Natural predators were used. Ladybugs killed unwelcome insects. Ironically, the pesticides kill the ladybugs. Cats were used to dispose of rodents. When natural methods were used, cancer rates were lower. We are losing the war on cancer. Our chemicalized water, air, food, drugs and cosmetics are killing us. A glaring example: Before Dioxin, it was assumed that one of the five Americans would get cancer. After Dioxin, it is assumed that one of three will.

What harm, besides cancer, results when pesticides pollute the water? Birth defects, central nervous system illness, reproductive problems can result. As the use of pesticides increased, so did the contamination of our water.

Pesticide poisoning is not just common in farmland. Home pesticide use increases the incidence of leukemia in children. Lawn care sprays are dangerous. Flea powders, weed sprays and mothballs are dangerous.

A list of the dangerous pesticides used for non-agricultural purposes is printed in a book called "Drinking Water Hazards."

Waste with human afflictions, circumstantial evidence makes our waste streams suspect.

The Mississippi River collects an abundant wasteland on the way to the sea. Parts of Louisiana use it for drinking water. Those that do, experience statistically significant higher rates of cancer than those who do not.

I refer to total cancer. Cancer of the urinary organs and cancer of the gastro-intestinal tract. From 1946 – 1970, the United States dumped low level radioactive waste offshore in steel drums at four sites in the Atlantic and two in the Pacific. Some radioactive waste has also leaked from defense sites and washed downstream. A moratorium now exists – on disposal at sea.

Various government agencies are responsible for safeguarding the health and lives of the citizens.

The contamination of our water from industrial chemical waste and pesticides is a major disaster. The citizens are plagued by cancer, nervous disorders, kidney problems, and birth defects because of this contamination.

Add to this scandal, the contamination of our water by the military and you have the citizens of our country deprived of ... their legal and moral right to safe drinking water.

The EPA's superfnd cleanup list includes names of military dumps and landfills, which contain explosives, chemicals, paints, and hazardous waste. The chemical PCB (polychlorinated Biphenyls), is dumped and is responsible for cancer and other devastating sickness and suffering.

The D.O.E. (Department of Energy) - a government agency, dumps waste that has radioactivity. This agency has contaminated thousands of ponds and water sites; so has the Department of Defense.

Who will defend us from our defenders? The government agencies cannot be regulated like private industry. They make their own rules. **They decide what pollution is**.

President Ronald Reagan signed an executive order, which allowed the Defense Department to clean up its own toxic sites. The Department of Energy, likewise, decides its own environmental policies. How can citizens fight such total ruthless disregard of their rights?

The first step is to demand information about the contamination. Knowledge is power. State and Federal legislators should be bombarded by letters from citizens, demanding that they be kept informed.

State and Federal legislators should be bombarded by letters from citizens demanding that the D.O.E. and DOD be subject to Federal Laws and be regulated by the EPA

When oil, chemicals, radioactive waste and other deadly contaminents are found in a community's water supply, the people should file Class Action Lawsuits against the industry of the military outfit that is poisoning their water.

The pollution of the nation's drinking water comes from many sources. The water treatment plants can pollute water by the over use of chlorine.

The pipes used to transport water can be dangerous. Plastic pipes made with Polyvinyl Chloride (PVC) use chemical glue to join the sections of the pipe.

Gasoline and pesticides from contaminated groundwater pass through plastic pipes. Chemicals permeate plastic pipes so readily that such pipes should not be used where there is already contamination of the land and the water.

Copper pipes allow practically no contamination of cancer causing chemicals. They should be used. In cancer, as in other diseases, an ounce of prevention is worth a pound of cure.

The agency responsible for clean water and air is the EPA. This stands for Environmental Protection Agency. Its performance suggests that some of its personnel think it stands for - 'Every Poison Allowed'.

The effort to clean water costs billions. It must be made. Water is life. Water pollution is death. A clean-up effort will be met with opposition.

Chemicals are a one hundred million dollar a year business. The Chemical Manufacturers Association is the trade association for this industry. It fights efforts to curb and control pollution.

In December 1970, the Environmental Protection Agency was formed to control national problems of crisis proportions – disposal of toxic waste, clean up of waterways and air.

Congress called for a report by the EPA on the agency's efforts to address the problem. This report was not given until 1975. Obviously, the agency failed to meet its obligations.

For a few years in the 1970's, the EPA tried to regulate the disposal of toxic waste and begin a clean up of water and air. The agency is the largest regulatory agency in the government.

It is grossly under-funded. It deals with many political and economic groups, Congress, state officials, industrial, and the public. It needs more money than it is allotted, to do its work.

Still, the bureaucracy suffers from more than a lack of financial resources. It is an indecisive, sluggish agency, lacking men and women who are dedicated to enforcing laws passed to protect the people.

An example of bureaucratic foot dragging is the failure to enforce the Safe Drinking Law passed in December of 1974. The EPA had empowerment to enforce standards for hazardous substances found in drinking water.

In the first ten years after the act was passed the EPA only sent twenty-one cases of violation to the Justice Department for prosecution.

Thousands of violations occur each year. This is a very serious failure.

Wilhelm Huepner was head of the National Cancer Institute in Environmental Cancer section in the 1960's. He said, "The rapidly increasing pollution of many bodies of fresh and salt water with carcinogenic agents and the inabilities of the presently used filtration equipment to remove such contaminants from the drinking water supply have created conditions that may result in serious cancer hazards to the general population.

The non-enforcement by the EPA of the Safe Water Act led to the filing of the lawsuits against that agency by citizens interested in the environment. The tax payers had to try to teach the EPA bureaucrats how to do their job.

The EPA has suggested setting standards for nine toxic chemicals that show up in groundwater: TCE, vinyl chloride, benzene, PCE, carbon tetrachloride, L, 1 dichcoro ethane, L, 2 dichloroethylene and dichlorogenze. Seven of these are considered carcinogens.

There are many hundreds more contaminants of drinking water than the nine listed. Some of them are: mercury, lead, cadmium, arsenic, asbestos, chromium, nitrates, dioxin, aldicarb – to name a few!

These poisons unregulated are dumped into our water and land. They cause, in addition to cancer, kidney problems, skin rashes, respiratory defects. Is it any wonder that American citizens are plagued with so much serious sickness?

The EPA sets standards which it does not enforce. In 1978, Congress passed the Uranium Mill Tailings Radiation Control Act. This act gave the EPA a May 1980 deadline for establishing health and safety standards for mill tailings.

After EPA established them, the Nuclear Regulatory Commission would make regulations to implement them. What happened? The EPA stalled. In October of 1980, the NRC proceeded to implement regulations from guidelines they thought the EPA should have set. The NRC wanted to set limitations on the level of radioactivity that mill tailings could emit. The NRC ordered that mill tailings be covered with rock and earth.

Three years later, in September of 1983, the EPA finally announced it had set standards to restrict emissions from mill tailings, and to restrict their seepage into groundwater.

These standards permitted radiation releases ten times greater than the standards the NRC had suggested. So much for any protection from radioactivity that the tax paying citizens could have expected.

Although the EPA has concentrated surface water clean up, groundwater has become more hazardous, as evidenced by the Love Canal incident.

The EPA, responsible for the clean-up of hazardous waste sites, needed money for its monumental task. In 1980, legislation was passed. The comprehensive Environmental Response Compensation and Liability Act of 1980 is often called the Superfund Act.

This law holds the parties who dumped hazardous waste responsible for its clean-up. When the responsible parties cannot be located or refuse to clean up, the money for the clean up comes from a special fund established for that purpose.

The use of the Superfund by the EPA was sluggish. The entire performance of the EPA, since it was established in December of 1970, has been sluggish. In 1972 the Federal Insecticides, Fungecide and Rodenticide Act became law. It mandated that new products should be

69

submitted by the manufacturers to the EPA for Safety Tests - old products should re-register for inspection.

The EPA spent five years studying Toxaphene, a pesticide which causes cancer, before restricting it. And the incidence of cancer in our country continues to increase.

The EPA "consults" with the Chemical Industries. While the government employees are 'meeting' with the industries executives, dangerous chemicals REMAIN IN USE! No such 'joint studies' should be permitted.

As a matter of fact, dangerous chemical products should not be allowed on the market. A new product should be proven safe BEFORE given permission for sale to the public.

Tests for carcinogenicity and tetragewicity should be done on animals. Why should tax payers play guinea pig? Why should tax payers use chemicals that cause cancer and birth defects for years, while the EPA 'studies' them?

The tragic consequences of allowing use of dangerous chemicals are magnified by the fact that once these chemicals seep into the groundwater THEY STAY THERE. Some chemicals dissipate after years. Some remain FOREVER.

The Chemical Manufacturers Association (C.M.A.) is a trade association which wields too much power. The chemical industry nets billions of dollars annually. No member of C.M.A. should be allowed to 'study' with an employee of the EPA

States must test water quality so it meets federal requirements.

Enforce EPA standards as set forth in Safe Drinking Water Act.

When states fail to test water and the citizens suspect dangerous levels of radioactivity and chemicals, and pesticides, the citizens should notify the EPA

Citizen involvement is an absolute MUST if water is to be made safe. The interests of public health are not considered by Agribusiness, the steel, rubber, oil, chemical industries, or by the government agencies which are supposed to regulate them.

CHAPTER TEN

The Air We Breathe

The United States of America is considered a wealthy country. Other nations speak enviously of our wealth. However, some of the nation's wealth has been and is still being generated at the expense of the citizens' health and lives.

The technology that has brought prosperity is out of control. This technology has contaminated whole communities. It has damaged the Ozone Shield. It has released chloro-fluoro carbons into the air.

This technology has caused environmental damage with resultant environmental illnesses. Leukemia has increased. Skin cancer has increased. The odds that an American citizen will get cancer have increased. Before Dioxin, it was assumed that one in five would get cancer. Now it is one in three.

This is tragic. Is the economic growth that increases cancer acceptable? Air pollution as a cause of cancer has not been given enough attention – and regulation. Must we accept the pollution of our air, water, food – as essential to economic prosperity?

Of the thousands of toxic chemicals that pollute our air, only six have been given much attention. They are: Carbon Monoxide, Sulfur Dioxide, Particulates, Nitrogen Oxide, and Lead.

Federal laws have not addressed the problems caused by pollutants in the air.

The acceptance of pollution is based on a naïve assumption that we can clean it up. The incidents at Love Canal and Chernobyl should have told us that this is not the scenario.

We have assumed that others are responsible for pollution. At the same time we are spraying lawns, and crops with deadly poisons that linger. We use products, the making of which, increase pollution.

Bureaucracies cannot "clean it up". Industrial groups lobby against government activities to impose regulations.

Actually, human beings cannot regulate nature. We must understand that we are making a bad impact on nature when we spew toxic fumes in the air. We must understand that our land cannot be used as a dump for toxic matter.

The poisonous products that technology has created are not disposed of the way we assumed they would be. Products like Phenylphenol do not just disappear. Phenol has been combined with chlorine to form products called chlorophenols. These are used in weed killers, and in products to prevent mold and fungus in wood, etc.

The next development was Trichlorophenol – used in herbicides, like 24D and 24ST in Vietnam. This product was called "Agent Orange". The protests about this product were first made by Vietnam Ware Veterans who claimed they caused cancer and birth defects.

A new compound formed during the manufacture of Trichlorophenol was called 2378TCDD – It is known as Dioxin. It is the most toxic synthetic chemical known to man. It created the disaster at Love Canal.

TCDD – Dioxin – has been researched in EPA laboratories. It was found to be more toxic than cyanide. Animal studies proved that Dioxin can have adverse effects on any organ in the body. It is a carcinogen of such potency that it is without precedent.

In addition to being carcinogenic, Dioxin is teratogenic (causing birth defects). It was reported that in Soueso, Italy, in 1976, Dioxin was accidentally released. The people exposed had chloracne, spontanious abortions, and birth defects, like Spina Bifida and Polydactyl – (too many toes and fingers).

In 1973 the danger of chlorofluorcarbons (C.F.C.'s) was discovered. It was not acknowledged until 1987.

When scientists, who were concerned that these C.F.C.'s caused a hole in the ozone over the Antarctic tried to warn of the danger, the chemical companies tried to discredit them.

The C.F.C. industry was an eight billion dollar a year industry. One million tons of C.F.C. were polluting the atmosphere. This is unacceptable. Russell Peterson, former Chairman of President's Council on Environmental Quality said, "We cannot afford to give chemicals the same constitutional rights that we enjoy under the law. Chemicals are not innocent until proven guilty.

The United States has the leadership in the field of industrial chemicals. When the hole in the ozone layer was traced to C.F.C.'s there was great concern about jobs being lost. It was claimed that thousands of jobs would be lost if C.F.C's were banned.

People asked what would happen if the jobs were lost and then it was discovered that the greenhouse effect was absorbed by natural planetary weather systems and the oceans.

There are several wrong assumptions behind this reasoning:

1. Chemicals are guilty until proven innocent.

2. If the chemical is used until proven innocent beyond a reasonable doubt – but is found to be guilty – the damage to the ozone cannot be reversed. It is permanent.

3. Dead men and women do not need jobs.

In spite of the discovery that C.F.C.'s were creating a hole in the ozone, the EPA refused to ban C.F.C.'s in 1984. Half of the ozone: over 12.5 million miles of land and sea has been destroyed. The full implications of this will not be known for years.

BIBLIOGRAPHY

1. "The Body is the Hero", Ronald J. Glasser, Random House, 1976
2. "The Conquest of Cancer", Dr. Virginia Livingston-Wheeler and Edmond G. Addeo, Franklin Watts, 387 Park Ave., New York, NY 10016.
3. "Radiation, What It Is, How It Affects You", Jack Schubert, Ralph E. Lapp, The Viking Press, 625 Madison Avenue, New York, NY 10957.
4. "At High Risk", Christopher Norwood, Mc Graw Hill, New York, NY
5. "The Chemical Feast", The Nader Report, James S. Turner, Grossman Publishers, 125 East 19th St., New York, NY 10003
6. "Vitamin B17 – Forbidden Weapon Against Cancer", Michael L. Culbert, Arlington House Publishers, New Rochelle, NY 10974

74

CHAPTER ELEVEN

An Ounce Of Prevention

There is one and only one sure cure for cancer – DO NOT GET IT! The only medicine of value in cancer, as in other diseases, is preventive medicine.

Articles in newspapers and announcements on T.V. newscasts have proclaimed that every effort is being made to find a cure for cancer. The field of immunotherapy is held out as a great promise. Hope is held out that immunotherapists will develop a vaccine.

Meanwhile, the news is grim. The harsh reality is that the rate of cancer has increased. The General Accounting Office (G.A.O.) has announced that no progress has been made in either reducing breast cancer or reducing the death rate from it.

More women are being diagnosed with breast cancer now than twenty years ago according to the GAO report to the House Government Committee on Human Services.

Richard Linster, GAO Auditor, said that there is now some optimism because of earlier diagnosis of breast tumors. However, the high death rate persists. "no inroads have been made in reducing the morality from the disease," according to Linster.

This year 175,000 American women will be diagnosed with breast cancer. Forty-five thousand will die of it. One in nine women will be diagnosed with breast cancer. Linster said, "Until we have a better understanding of the factors that cause breast cancer, efforts to prevent the disease have little chance of success."

The Environmental Protection Agency (EPA) has to enforce the laws it has not been enforcing. The technical and engineering expertise to the use of air pollution control equipment has been developed in Germany. The EPA would do well to learn more about this. Right now much of the air pollution control equipment in this country has been imported from Germany.

Another government agency that has failed to safeguard the safety of the citizens is the Atomic Energy Commission (A.E.C.). This powerful agency was supposed to promote the use of nuclear power for peaceful purposes.

Whole communities have been contaminated... The Dow Chemical Company pumped 300,000 gallons a day of chemicals into the ground for thirty years in Midland, Michigan. People now have symptons of Dioxin poisoning.

In Woburn, Massachusetts, industrial solvents contaminated groundwater. A high incidence of childhood leukemia resulted.

The government bought the town of Times Beach, Missouri, after a waste hauler, Russell Bliss, used Dioxin-polluted oil... to treat roads there and many other incidents. There will continue to be contamination of entire communities unless citizens organize and demand their rights.

The citizens pay the salaries of the men and women who work in the government agencies. The citizens must 'watch-dog' these agencies because it is painfully clear that said agencies have been corrupt. Their sins of omission and commission are responsible for threat. In the 1980's, the U.S. Environmental Protection Agency warned about Radon as a major cause of lung cancer.

Dr. Charles Dudney, a Radon researcher at Oak Ridge Tennessee National Laboratory, believes American people should become more knowledgeable about Radon. He also believes the administration during the 1980's failed to provide money for research and testing. The Radon research program at Oak Ridge is now almost inactive. Radon is a major cause of cancer.

The government should provide low cost or low interest loans to finance testing and modification of homes. The test costs about $25.00. American taxpayers should demand action on this program.

Better living through chemistry is a vicious canard. Shorter life span through chemistry is more realistic. More about this later.

The problem of clean air is vexing the environmental scientists. The threat of global warming and ozone depletion is under study, but proposals on how to handle the crisis are "science fiction" according to F. Sherwood Rowland of the University of California. He added, "Nothing proposed yet is remotely feasible."

James Hansen of NASA's Goddard Institute for Space Studies had an even bleaker assessment of scientific knowledge about environmental problems. He claimed that he and his colleagues "don't understand how we are changing the climate now." He warned that using unproven methods to reverse the damage already done could cause more problems than ones being solved.

Holes in the ozone layer in the spring season in Southern Chile have caused health problems, which were thought to be in the future. Skin cancer and blindness from unfiltered ultraviolet rays have increased in areas of the Southern Hemisphere.

How to prevent this alarming deterioration? Former Interior Secretary Donald Hodel suggested people wear hats, sunglasses, and a lot of sunscreen until we learn how a more useful preventive program would be. We should cut back on the burning of fossil fuels and stop using the chlorofluorcarbons that deplete the ozone layer.

These practices do not hold a solution. They will help us slow down the rate at which we are degrading the environment. But we must find better ways to try to reverse the damage we have inflicted on the environment. It is later than we think.

God created the Earth in perfect ecological balance. He gave us clean air, pure water, wholesome food. The polluters might be wise to remember God will not be mocked.

Cancer prevention techniques are available now. A way to lessen the risk of colon cancer is to eat a high fiber diet. To lower the risk of oral cancer, use betacarotene and Vitamin A. Pre-cancerous mouth lesions should be seen by a doctor or dentist who can supervise the use of the two nutrients.

Investigators at the National Cancer Institute reported on a mouthwash study they conducted. The risk of oral cancer jumped 90% in men who had used a mouthwash with high alcohol content. The report stated that this was true only of mouthwashes with 25% alcohol content.

Listerine is the only mouthwash with this content. The makers of Listerine, Warner-Lambert said they plan to market a mouthwash with lower alcohol content.

Dr. William Blot, one of the Authors of the study said, "Smoking and alcohol consumption are the two greatest and best established risk factors for the disease". Chewing tobacco is another factor.

Thirty-thousand new cases of oral cancer were diagnosed in the

U.S.A. in 1990. Early treatment has a 75% survival rate. Dark green, yellow or orange vegetables and fruits contain beta-carotene, which is cancer preventive.

Mothers who nursed their babies are at lower risk of breast cancer. Some experts suspect that estrogen replacement therapy and the birth control pill may be escalating the rate of breast cancer.

Breast implants have not been proven safe. The implants that have been covered with polyurethane foam release a chemical called Toluene Diamene or T.D.A., which is a carcinogen. Dr. David Black of Vanderbilt University, a toxicologist, is President of Aegis Analytical Corp. This is a drug testing company located in Nashville, Tennessee. He stated in his findings that the T.D.A. is found in small amounts in the milk of nursing mothers.

He believes it is a minor hazard to infants and that the hazard is greater to the woman who has the implant. When the finding was released, Sibyl Goldrich said, "The word is out." She is founder of Command Trust Network, a group devoted to the problems of implant patients. She added, "We kept waiting for the F.D.A. to announce something. But they never did."

A study in Sweden in 1989 showed that women who took estrogen had twice the rate of breast cancer as those who did not take hormones. Women who took that type of estrogen plus a progestin for four or more years had a rate of breast cancer four times that of women who took no hormones.

Dr. Robert Hoover, M.D., PhD, Chief of Environmental Epidemiology Branch of The National Cancer Institute, said, "This study adds to the body of evidence that long term use of menopausal replacement hormones increases a woman's risk of breast cancer."

In the spring of 1991, researchers from the Centers for Disease Control and Emory University, compared data. They believed the risk starts to increase after five years of estrogen therapy. It increases 30% after 15 years. This increase represents a large number of preventable breast cancer cases.

A new drug, tamoxifen, may prevent cancer of the breast. It is used in cancer treatment now. It has reduced mortality from a first breast tumor by 20%. A five year study is going on now to determine if tamoxifen tablets are a preventative measure.

At New York's Institute for Hormone Research, scientists have discovered an ingredient in cruciferous vegetables that might protect against cancer. Cruciferous vegetables are the cabbage family. This ingredient is called indole 3 carbinol. It causes estrogen to break down into inactive byproducts. It is the active products of estrogen that promote tumors. It is not established how much indole 3 carbinol is needed in the daily diet.

A new type of anti-cancer therapy called "biological therapy" is on the horizon. Vitamin A derivatives called retinoids have demonstrated ability to convert cancer cells into normal ones. At present, this is experimental and is used on advanced cases.

A drug derived from the yew tree, taxol, has shown an ability to shrink tumors.

A high fat diet can contribute to breast cancer link. A high fat diet contributes to the risk of any cancer. To lower your fat intake, eat leaner cuts of meat. Do not consume meat droppings. Meat contains zinc, iron, and B vitamins. If you stop eating red meat, you have to find foods with iron. Beans and grain products, when eaten together, are a source of iron.

Which meat has the most fat? Chicken drumstick, round bottom beef roast, pork loin chop, head the list. The least fat is in chicken breast, pork loin and beef eye round. Veal has the absolute lowest fat content, but I neither eat it or recommend it because of the extremely cruel treatment of the animals to produce veal.

Helpless calves are taken when a few days old and chained in a stall so small, movement is impossible. It is dark. Their joints swell. After about 15 weeks of torture, they die and are "tender veal". I will not subsidize this cruelty.

These fat contents of meat and poultry, by gram, were calculated for three ounce portions of cooked meat: Chicken drumstick with skin – 9.5 grams; beef bottom round – 7.4; pork loin center chop – 6.9; chicken breast with skin – 6.6; pork sirloin chop – 5.7; beef tip round – 5.4; lamb foreshank – 5.1; beef top round – 4.9; chicken drumstick without skin – 4.8; chicken breast without skin – 3.0; veal top round – 2.9.

It has been estimated that 70% of the cancer in the U.S.A. is preventable. It is a tragic waste of human life. Tragic, because methods of preventing cancer have not been studied and pursued. Tragic, because the methods now known are not common knowledge.

The single most important way to prevent cancer is to remove the carcinogens from our food, drugs and cosmetics. We use them daily and they are saturated with chemicals. It is important that air quality be improved. It is important that smoking become obsolete. But above all, we must clean up the food supply.

There are over six thousand chemical additives in our food. It would be impossible for the citizens to learn the name of each one. The most commonly used and potent ones can be identified and boycotted. These are: All artificial colors, artificial flavors, sodium nitrite and sodium nitrate. Books that identify other carcinogens will be listed. It is important that consumers read labels. It is vital that consumers write to the companies using carcinogens that they will not buy their products. Boycott!

Why has our food become so polluted and poisoned? The "Baby Boomers" of the 1940's and 1950's wanted new food products that could be used in a hurry. They wanted convenience food. Processed food became popular. Not only did the consumers get quick fix foods – the food industry discovered that the shelf life of their products was increased.

Problems with convenient processed food soon became obvious. The food did not taste fresh. The food was not health-giving. The minerals and vitamins had been lost in processing. The food had become empty calories. Then the problem of carcinogenicity become became obvious. Preservatives and chemical additives were found to cause cancer in tests on laboratory animals.

Humans are not members of the mineral kingdom. We are members of the animal kingdom. If a chemical food additive causes cancer in laboratory animals, I do not use it in my food. Period.

People are learning that the game is not worth the candle. They are asking for organic natural food. Jerry Cash, Professor of Food Science and Human Nutrition at Michigan State University, has predicted an increased interest in foods from organic crops. Such foods are considered healthier by consumers.

According to Mr. Cash, new foods will be "foodaceuticals". That is the term for new foods that focus on health. Between 1989 and 1990, the sales of foods labeled "all natural" increased by 175%. Obviously, consumes want to follow a cancer-preventive diet.

It is wise to read the ingredients on the label. I read a box that said "All Natural" but listed in the ingredients was carrageenan. It is an additive to be avoided.

The cancer preventive diet excluded use of aflatoxins. They are

80

poisons secreted by strains of the mold aspergillus flavusoryzae. These molds grow on wheat, rice, corn, and other grains when they are stored in humid conditions. Aflatoxins, like other carcinogens, are more dangerous when taken over a long period of time in very small amounts. Small amounts of carcinogens in our air, food, water, drugs and cosmetics are cancer-causing health hazards. The F.D.A. can allow minute doses of carcinogens with smug assurances they are "safe". I am not buying their story. Liver cancer is linked to aflatoxins in peanuts in some areas. To eliminate aflatoxins from our diet, changes must be made in the way that nuts and grains are harvested and stored. Such changes could help reduce and prevent cancer.

The cancer preventive diet is a low fat, high fiber diet. Fat substitutes are being developed. Complex carbohydrates can fill in for fat. Corn starch, maltodextrins, oat fiber are good. Synthetic fats have not been proven safe yet.

Fiber is an absolute must in a cancer preventive diet. Adequate fiber reduces the risk of cancer and heart disease; the major killers. Research has proven this. It is important to eat oat bran muffins and oat cereal, celery, carrots, potato skins, bananas, brussells sprouts, brown rice, whole wheat bread. About 20-35 grams of fiber per day is considered a high fiber diet. If you do not like vegetables, learn to like them. It is your life span.

The average American eats too much protein and only about eleven grams of fiber each day. Years ago, people ate more fiber. We moderns should increase our intake. We can start by having cereals every morning. The side panel of cereal boxes lists fiber content. I enjoy shredded wheat and Grape Nuts.

For those not interested in counting grams, it is sufficient to eat enough fruits, vegetables, cereals and bread every day. All fruits and vegetables, cereals and bread every day. All fruits and vegetables should be soaked in water to remove the pesticides.

Instead of orange juice, eat the orange. Instead of instant mashed potatoes, eat the whole potato – with the skin. The insoluble part of wheat bran is thought to reduce risk of cancer in the colon. When eating a high fiber diet it is very important to drink at least eight glasses of water every day.

A low fat diet can reduce the risk of getting cancer. A low fat diet brings benefits other than reducing the risk of cancer. It is a good source of energy. It has a cosmetic value as it helps maintain a lower weight.

Will it be tasty? This is important. We want to stay on it – and we have a right to enjoy eating. There are fat-burning food that are tasty.

Bread is a food for all seasons. It introduces fiber into the diet and decreases fat. It also adds the important carbohydrates. Tasty breads like rye, pumpernickel, Russian black bread offer variety. Banana bread is a treat.

The United States Department of Agriculture has recommended that we eat fruit and vegetables every day. We are advised to eat from three to five vegetables and from two to four servings of fruit daily.

These fat-burning foods contain vitamins and minerals essential for good health. Potatoes have twice as much Potassium – a mineral which allays fluid retention – as bananas. Most of it is in the skin. Potatoes are maligned as fattening, but the potato is not guilty. The sauces and creams added to it are guilty.

Bananas have more than fiber to recommend them. They are high in Potassium and Vitamin C. They contain enough sugar in the form of Fructose to satisfy a sweet tooth.

In order to get variety in a diet full of vegetables and fruit, we should discover the global food market. New food tastes are there to be discovered and enjoyed. For example, we just discussed the banana. The red banana is sweeter than the yellow one and just as rich in Vitamin C. Plantains can be yellow or green. They contain two important minerals: Potassium and Niacin.

Passion fruit is a lemony, tart tasting fruit which enhances any fruit salad. Chayote is a delicious food which tastes like a combination of apple and cucumber. Tamaring is a pod which can be pureed. Its pulp has a flavor of apricots and dates.

The cactus pear, which is available from July to March, can be peeled, seeded, then pureed to make yogurt. With a flavor similar to watermelon, it is rich in Potassium and Vitamin C.

The horned melon is rich in Potassium and Vitamin C. It tastes like a combination of cucumber, banana and lime. Chestnuts are low in fat. A cup of roasted chestnuts has three grams of fat, while a cup of walnuts or almonds has 25 times that amount. Chestnuts are rich in Potassium and Vitamin C and B. They should be hard, shiny brown and feel heavy.

To roast them, just cut an X in the flat side of the shell, then bake about fifteen minutes at 400 degrees F. Sweet potatoes and chestnuts can be baked together with brown sugar and margarine. Peeled, chopped, roasted chestnuts can be baked with oranges and cranberries into a bread which is delicious, different and healthy.

Exotic foods, in addition to giving nutritional benefits, enhance an otherwise boring steady diet of foods we have eaten all of our lives.

Dr. Virginia Livingston, cancer researcher, discovered that Abscisic acid is an anti-cancer agent. Foods that contain it are:

FOODS CONTAINING ABSCISIC ACID

FRUITSROOT VEGETABLES
MangosAll – Especially Carrots
Grapes
Avocados
Pears*SEEDS AND NUTS*
OrangesOf all kinds
Apples with seeds

FRUIT BLOSSOMS AND LEAVES AS TEALEAFY VEGETABLES
Peach flowersOf all kinds
Strawberry / leaves
Cherry flowers
Apple Blossoms

ALL SEEDS, NUTS, ROOT STORAGE
VEGETABLES WITH MATURE GREENS

VEGETABLES
Pea shoots
Lima beans
Potatoes
Peas, dwarf
Yams
Sweet potatoes
Asparagus

Tomatoes
Onions
Spinach

A major study by the American Cancer Society revealed preliminary evidence that aspirin reduces the risk of cancer of the colon. Aspirin (Acetylsalicylic acid) interferes with production of prostaglandins. One prostoglandin plays a role in cell proliferation. Thus, aspirin may inhibit the cell proliferation of cancer and reduce the risk of cancer. Too much aspirin can be risky. The most successful cancer prevention lifestyle involves not smoking, eating the low fat, high fiber diet and avoiding what Ralph Nader called, "The Chemical Feast."

Cancer prevention includes improvement in air quality in the home as well as the great outdoors. Homes should be well ventilated. A garage should be aired out to reduce carbon monoxide, nitrogen dioxide, and other products of exhaust systems. They can float into the house.

Pesticides, paint, paint thinners, etc., exude a gaseous stream of volatile organic compounds – VOC's. Such items should not be kept in a garage. They belong outside. Fiberboard cabinets can seep Formaldehyde. Cleansers and polishes can exude VOCS's. Flea bombs can pollute the air. To improve air quality in your home, reduce the use of chemical sprays.

Chemical Manufactures Association, 2501 M St., NW, Washington, D.C. 20037.

Cosmetic Toiletry and Fragrance Association, 1110 Vermont Ave., NW, Suite 800, Washington, DC 20005

Grocery Manufacturers of America, 1010 Wisconsin Ave., NW, Suite 800, Washington, DC 20007

National Confectioners Association of the USA, 7900 West Park Dr., Suite A-320, McLean, VA 22102

National Food Processors Association, 1401 New York Ave. NW, 4th Fl., Washington, DC 20005

Snack Food Association, 1711 King St., Suite 1, Alexandria, VA 22314

The names of more trade associations are listed in "The Encyclopedia of Associations". This is available in the reference room of most public libraries. It is published by: Gale Research, Inc., PO Box 441914, Detroit, MI 48244.

CHAPTER TWELVE

Fight Back

Beleagured and betrayed, American consumers can fight back. There are ways. First, they have to wake up and smell, not the coffee, but the odor of corruption and greed. Corruption is government agencies which are supposed to safeguard their health. Greed from agribusiness and the pharmaceutical companies.

We must get angry. We must write angry letters to our legislators and demand action. We must inform them that we want the Delaney Amendments enforced. Congressman, James Delaney of New York fought long and hard to get his Amendment into law. One of his opponents was the A.M.A.

We must demand the abolition of the F.D.A. which has had since 1958, to enforce this law. A new agency, independent of agribusiness and drug cartels, should be formed with a new staff.

We must insist that scientists who work for government agencies stop holding conflict of interest jobs. One member of the National Academy of Science was also on the payroll of three drug companies. The N.A.S. has to be relieved of its duties as a deciding arm of the F.D.A.

Your Congressman or Congresswoman is elected. Write him or her that you are studying their responses to your demands. Congressional committees are now in existence for the purpose of consumer protection. Lobby them. There is a Consumer Subcommittee of the Committee on Commerce. There is an Intergovernmental Relations Subcommittee of the Committee on Governmental Operations.

The people who are making decisions about products that can cause cancer, birth defects and other diseases, must be held

86

accountable for their decisions. Alibis cannot be accepted. "I was just doing what I was told" is not an excuse. "It's just a small amount of sodium nitrite" is not an excuse.

"There are natural Carcinogens in food" is not an excuse. There are natural carcinogens. Corn, wheat, and peanut butter are aflatoxins which are carcinogenic. But that is no reason to add chemical carcinogens to food.

Vitamins C and E are cancer Preventive. So is Beta Carotene which contains Vitamin A. Certain foods like carrots and asparagus are cancer preventive. Has any government agency published a booklet listing these foods?

Lobbying Congress is important. However, it takes time. We are out of time in the war on cancer. The fastest way to clean up our food and drug supply is to BOYCOTT!

We must inform the food industry we will not buy their products unless they remove the additives. Additives are not there for our benefit. They have no nutritional value. They are to increase shelf life of the product. "Anything for a buck" is the motto of these people.

We must write to the trade associations. At the end of this chapter is a partial list of places to write. It is vitally important to talk to the managers of food stores where we shop. Notify them you will not buy a specific item. For example, "I have shopped at your store a long time. I will not buy any more of product X because it contains yellow dye No. 5, which is a potent carcinogen. I am telling my friends and neighbors to boycott this product." The store manager is probably as uninformed about the product as you were. He is in business to make a profit. If an item cannot be moved, he will not reorder it. Soon, the food manufacturer will get the message. He will remove the dangerous additive for business reasons – where he would not remove it for the consumers' health.

It is impossible to appeal to a sense of decency or honesty, because the people who polluted our food have none. They have bribed. They have pressured the F.D.A. to keep their dangerous additives in use. They have NO social conscience. All they understand is profit and loss.

They do not use their own deadly products. I talked to a chemist who developed a frequently used additive. He told me he never uses any food products. I talked to a chemist who developed a frequently used additive. He told me he never uses any food product which contains the chemical additive he developed. Right from the horse's mouth!!

Here with is a sampling of letters which can be used to base your own campaign of protest to manufacturers of these products and your congressional representatives:

OPEN LETTER TO THE EDITORS
OF "PREVENTION" MAGAZINE

Prevention
P.O. Box 182
Emmaus, PA 18099

Dear Editors:

With shock and dismay, I read that you have approved of irradiation of food. What do you know about the potential threat to the health and life of humans who eat irradiated food?

Have you any legitmate basis for stating that it is "safe"? Are you aware that Dr. John Gofman, a world-reknowned authority on low level irradiation, said that research on the safety of irradiation has never been done? He stated that such a study will not be done because, ". . . It would require controlling the diets of at least 200,000 humans of various age groups for at least thirty years and following their health histories for at least fifty years (preferably their full lifespans)".

Are you aware that laboratory mice who were fed irradiated food developed malignant tumors? Are you aware that irradiated foods reduce levels of Viamins C, E, A and B complex?

Do you know why there is a campaign to irradiate our food? Billions of dollars will be made by the ruthless people who sell Cobalt 60 and Cesium 137 used in irradiation.

I am asking you to reverse your position. Please make a public statement that you are withdrawing your approval of irradiation.

Thank you.
Sincerely,

LETTERS TO FOOD CORPORATIONS

Letters to food corporations are important. Here are a few examples:

Lykes Bros., Inc.
Plant City, FL 33567

To Whom it May Concern:

I read the label on your product "Family Favorite Luncheon Loaf." It contains Monosodium Glutamate, Sodium Nitrate, Sodium Erythorbate, Sodium Phosphate, salt.

Are you aware that Sodium Nitrate combines with amines in the human body to form Nitrosamines? Are you aware that Nitrosamines are powerful carcinogens? If not, why not? I will not buy your product and will urge my friends and acquaintances to boycott it also.

Sincerely,

Campbell's Soup Company
Camden, NJ 08103

To Whom it May Concern:

I read the label on your "Dinosaur Vegetable Soup". This product is presented to appeal to children. Ingredients include: Disodium Guanylate, Disodium Inosinate, Thiamine Mononitrate.

Are you aware that Nitrates and Nitrites are carcinogens? Are you aware of the increase in the rate of cancer in children? More and more children are being victimized by this painful, deadly disease.

You have soup on the market like your "Tomato Bisque" which does not contain such deadly additives. Please remove them from your

"Dinosaur Vegetable Soup".

Thank you.

Sincerely,

POSITIVE LETTERS TO MANUFACTURERS

I have written in a very negative way about the fact we live in a cancer culture. I have urged boycott and protest.

Now I want to urge positive measures. By the same token that we complain about the pollution of our air, food, drugs, we should write letters of commendation to the corporations when they make safe products. It is always good to encourage people who are doing good things. Herewith are two examples of letters praising the efforts of these companies:

Chun King Corporation
Cambridge, MD 21613

To Whom it May Concern:

Congratuations on your fine product "Bamboo Shoots". I was impressed when I read the label: "No preservatives, artificial colors, no artificial flavors". Just the bamboo shoots and water. It is good to know that your corporation has a conscience for the consumers.

In this time when cancer is on the increase, it is gratifying to know that honest people have developed a safe product.

Thank you.
Sincerely,

Ortega Refried beans
Nabisco Brands, Inc.
East Hanover, NJ 07936

To Whom it May Concern:

Congratuations on your fine product: "Ortega Refried Beans". Its ingredients are simply: Pinto beans, water, soybeans, salt, no artificial color, cotton seed. This product is safe and tasty. Is is very commendable of you to avoid using artificial colors. They are carcinogenic and are in the food supply illegally.

The Delaney Amendment (1958) to the Pure Food, Drugs, Cosmetics Act forbids the use of any chemical additives which are carcinogenic.

I will be happy to recommend your product.

Sincerely,

CHAPTER THIRTEEN

Out With The Old, In With The New

Although chemotherapy is an "old" accepted and "proven"? therapy, it is not a cure. It has never been proven to be safe. Chemotherapy drugs block a necessary metabolic step in the process of cell division. Cancer cells divide faster than normal cells. Thus the drugs used in chemotherapy are able to poison normal cells as well as cancer cells.

Furthermore, chemotherapy often devastates the immune system because it poisons the dividing cells of bone marrow which is the foundation of the immune system.

Once the immune system is devastated, the patient is open to deadly infections. Sometimes patients on chemotherapy die of infections while attempting to be cured of cancer. Some patients tolerate this treatment whereas others suffer projectile vomiting, baldness, toxic reactions which are severe. Some patients seem to recover then develop a new cancer a few years later. This is due to the fact that many of the drugs used in chemotherapy are carcinogens.

For a list of the drugs used in chemotherapy, you can consult pages 75 and 76 in a book which describes the drugs by trade name and common names. This list was researched and composed with the *Physicians Desk Reference* (P.D.R.) of 1988 as the main source.

According to the P.D.R., all drugs used in chemotherapy are poisonous. Two examples: Methotraxate can have fatal or severe toxic reactions. Interferon Alpha 28 is so toxic that patients are hospitalized in the intensive care unit so they can survive the treatment!

Since this painful therapy has not been proven a cure for cancer, why is it so widely used? Chemotherapy was a 200 million dollar a

92

year industry until the 1980's when the amount almost tripled.

The drug companies have powerful influence in cancer treatment centers and are advisers to the National Cancer Institute!

In recent years, almost every anti-cancer drug was patented by the manufacturer despite the fact that the research was done at government supported institutions. The taxpayers were exploited again. The consumers pay for development of chemical drugs then pay exorbitant prices when they buy them.

The outrageous profits of the pharmaceutical companies explain why there is a campaign to discredit every new non-toxic, inexpensive therapy for cancer. These therapies are worth investigation even if they do not cure. If they ease suffering and prolong survival time, they deserve support.

The incredible profits for the pharmaceutical companies also explain why there has been such emphasis on a "cure" for this dreaded disease, instead of a concerted effort to teach prevention. While profit margins rise, people die and the government agencies formed to regulate, are indifferent.

"New" therapies have been and are being developed in spite of and not because of assistance from the Sloan-Kettering Institute, the American Cancer Society, the National Cancer Institute. These therapies are condemned without trial after phony investigations by the F.D.A.

Alternative non-toxic therapies are quickly labeled as "quackery" by the F.D.A. and the A.C.S. with no honest investigation into their potential or their success records. The A.C.S. went so far as to publish a book about new unorthodox procedures and call this book "Unproven Methods of Cancer Management".

Although many of these new therapies were developed by medical doctors and honest, qualified scientists, these men and women were labeled as "quacks". No clinical double blind tests or studies were conducted on some of these therapies. They were dismissed out of hand.

This system perpetuates the financially rewarding position of the powerful American Cancer Society (A.C.S.) which gets millions of dollars from consumers in government grants while suppressing new therapies which hold promise of real help for cancer victims.

A glaring example of the vicious practice of dismissing new therapies is the way the A.C.S. reacted to a very important discovery by Dr. Virginia Livingston. In tests on animals, she discovered a natural substance in foods which has an anticancer effect. It is called Abscisic Acid. It resembles Vitamin A and is a strong anti-cancer agent.

It seems strange that the A.C.S. never announced this breakthrough. Instead, this agency listed Dr. Livingston's therapies in its book, "Unproven Methods of Cancer Management".

This is the same agency that touts chemotherapy which, by now, is suspect of causing cancer! It would benefit the human race if the A.C.S. would stop the pernicious practice of discrediting every promising new therapy.

It is though the field of immunology that a breakthrough will be realized. It will not come through surgery, radiation, or chemotherapy. The cut, burn, poison line of treatments will be replaced with treatments of the immune system.

Surgery cannot remove every malignant cell. It is absolutely necessary at times, but is not a definitive cure. Radiation can injure healthy cells and is not a definitive cure. Chemotherapy is not the final solution. The A.C.S. would do well to encourage developments in the field of immunology.

Foods containing Abscisic acid are fruits and vegetables. They are listed in the chapter "An Ounce of Prevention". Of course, I refer to fresh fruits and vegetables.

The mistreatment given to Dr. Livingston is not exceptional. It was endured by others who labored long and hard in efforts to understand and conquer the scourge of cancer.

Dr. Lawrence Burton extracted a tumor inhibiting factor in the 1950's. He worked in New York with Dr. Frank Friedman, Dr. Antonio Rottino, M.L. Kaplan, and Dr. Robert Kassel. They had research grants from the N.C.I. and the Damon Runyon Memorial Fund for Cancer Research.

This team extracted a factor from mouse blood that caused long term remission of cancer in mice. They worked at St. Vincent's Hospital. Cancers in mice disappeared! They returned later, but a relationship between normal blood and a defense against cancer had been established. What reaction was given this discovery? St. Vincent's cancelled the grant! Dr. Burton never claimed he had found a cure. He called it a "control".

He relocated to the Bahamas. The F.D.A., so often the enemy of the people, blocked the importation of his serum into the U.S.A. His immuno-augmentative therapy was denied recognition. Once again our government denied the citizens their right to choose an alternate therapy or even use it along side a conventional therapy.

Dr. Dean Burk, a biochemist, carried on the work of Otto Warburg who was a biochemist. According to Dr. Warburg, if a way could be found to stop this fermentation, cancer might be stopped.

Using this theory as a starting point, Dr. Joseph Gold assumed that the cause of death in cancer, cachexia,, could be controlled. He believed that cancer combusts glucose (sugar) an creates Lactic Acid as a waste product. This Lactic Acid reconverts to Glucose which fuels a tumor and depletes the body. Dr. Gold wanted to stop this process.

He used Hydrazine Sulfate to block an enzyme in the liver that allowed the Lactic Acid to convert to Glucose.

Dr. Burk encouraged Dr. Gold and said he considered Hydrazine Sulfate the best anti-cancer agent. Dr. Gold was working at the Syracuse Cancer Research Institute in New York. His treatment was used on 84 patients and 70% had improvement without the disastrous side effects of standard chemotherapy.

Dr. Gold rightly considered Hydrazine Sulfate a new type of non-toxic chemotherapy. This compound was INEXPENSIVE. It did not destroy bone marrow like standard chemotherapy. It opened new horizons for a safer, less expensive, more successful therapy for cancer.

What happened? Calbio Chem of California, once interested in Hydrazine Sulfate, lost interest. The A.C.S. put it on its list of unproven methods. Dr. Gold lost funding. He persisted in his work. He found support from Russian scientists who accepted his hypothesis that Hydrazine Sulfate attacks the growth of cancer cells.

The researchers at Leningrad's N.N. Petrov Research Institute of Oncology of the U.S.S.R. Ministry of Health endorsed Dr. Gold's belief in Hydrazine Sulfate. They agreed that it controlled Malignant growths in humans in a relatively non-toxic way.

Then, doctors in America showed interest. One conducted double blind studies and concluded Hydrazine Sulfate influenced survival. Although this agent was being used by more doctors and helped victims prolong their lives, it still was not given fair evaluation or approval by the American cancer establishment.

As a matter of fact, the F.D.A. raided two companies that distributed supplies of Hydrazine Sulfate and seized the drug as well as literature about it! This agency, which has failed to enforce laws banning carcinogens in our food, drugs, and cosmetics, wanted to be certain citizens were denied relief from the disease they were not trying to curb.

Dr. Gold has been denied funding. However, his work continues. His address is:

Dr. Joseph Gold
Syracuse Cancer Research Institute
Presidential Plaza
600 E. Genesee St.
Syracuse, NY 13202

Another new non-toxic therapy which deserves investigation is one developed by Dr. Linus Pauling. It involves the use of Vitamin C. This vitamin prevents the formation of Nitrosamine – a powerful carcinogen.

Dr. Pauling believes that Vitamin C can be incorporated in the use of immunotherapy as a treatment for cancer. The basic idea of immunotherapy is especially attractive because it involves fighting the disease by natural means. The body's own defense mechanisms are used. The danger of serious side effects from the treatment is accordingly small.

The idea of stimulating the immunoglobulins and lymphocytes to destroy tumors was utilized by Dr. William B. Coley. Dr. Coley was a surgeon in New York when he developed mixed toxins to stimulate the immune system.

Some of Dr. Coley's patients showed great improvement. About half of his patients recovered. But X-rays and Radium were discovered at this time. Dr. Coley's toxins, which stimulated the immune system, were ignored.

A new method of stimulating immune lympholytes to attack a tumor is to insure a high intake of Vitamin C and Vitamin A. Nutrition as part of a treatment for cancer was suggested by Dr. Max Gerson. He achieved results with a strict diet and detoxification program. Although not a cure, nutrition has value as a component in cancer treatment.

Richard Passwater, in his book "Cancer and its Nutritional Theories" found cancer patients have "lower than average amounts of Vitamin C in their blood plasma and white corpuscles."

Dr. Ewan Cameron at Vale of Leven District Hospital in Loch Lomond Side Scotland agreed with Dr. Pauling that cancer patients taking Vitamin C had a longer survival time. Patients taking 10 grams of Vitamin C daily, lived four times as long as patients who did not.

Man and the guinea pig do not synthesize Vitamin C. They must have a *daily* intake. This is vital because Vitamin C is vital to proper functioning of the immune system. All cancer patients have decreased effectiveness of their immune system.

Another blessing this Vitamin brings: Vitamin C leads to a larger production of Interferon. Evidence is now in that Interferon can help control a developing cancer. Vitamin C helps convert toxic substances into non-toxic derivatives which are eliminated in urine. It detoxifies cancer producing substances like the Nitrosamines.

It is important for Americans to keep Vitamin C levels adequate. Americans eat more nitrated and nitrated meat than any other people. These nitrates and nitrites combine with amines in the body to form Nitrosamines which are powerful carcinogens.

I am not suggesting Vitamin C is a cure for cancer. I am stating emphatically it helps the immune system fight cancer. It has a role in the prevention and treatment of cancer.

It can be taken along with conventional therapies. One of its great advantages in improving the general health of a cancer patient is that it does no harm. The same cannot be said of the chemicals used in chemotherapy.

Dr. E. Cheraskin, in 1968, reported that his cancer patients on radiation had a better response to treatment when given Vitamin C daily. These patients were given Vitamin C one week before treatment and three weeks after in daily doses of 750 mg.

During chemotherapy, Vitamin C should not be given. It can be given during intervals between intense treatment in a help to the immune system.

Anti-oxidants help protect against cancer. Vitamin E is an anti-oxidant. Two food additives are anti-oxidants: BHA (Butylated Hydroxyanisole) and BHT (Butylated Hydroxytollne). Dr. Lee W. Wattenberg of the University of Minnesota Medical School has reduced stomach tumors with them.

Tests have shown that Vitamin A inhibited carcinogens and virus induced cancers in laboratory animals. All vitamins should be taken carefully. You can get too much of a good thing! It is best to consult a doctor who understands nutrition as part of preventive medicine – if you can find one.

One nutritional approach to cancer was the use of Laetrile. This was obtained from apricot and almond seeds. They contain Cyanide, a substance that kills cancer cells.

Although laetrile was used on 3000,000 people and increased their survival time, it was opposed by the A.M.A., A.C.S and F.D.A. These agencies discard any natural method which improves general health and survival time.

They operate in a fantasy world on the assumption that some "magic bullet" cure will be discovered. Of course it will be costly.

Laetrile was never given a fair chance. Dr. Kanematsu Sugiura worked at Sloan Kettering for years. He stated, "I still think my experimental results on the effect of Amygdalin (with high doses) on spontaneous mammary tumors (Adenocarcinomas) are correct."

Stoppage of growth of small tumors temporarily prevents the development of lung metastases – 8% against 20%. In a control group, saline delayed the development of spontaneous cancers for three to four months.

We do not live in a democracy. We live in a corporate state. Our congress men and women have been bought and paid for by corporations. These corporations have fought to destroy the environmental protection agency.

When the E.P.A. tries to enforce laws like the clean water act – congress will not support the effort. We must write our congress men and women that we want these laws enforced.

Recently it was announced that a new promising treatment wipes out cancer in mice. Drugs called angiostatin and Endostatin are used.

This is an outrage. Why should we cheer a cure for mice? Twenty two years ago, Dr. Stanislaw Burzynski and Carlton Hazelwood were using antineoplastons to cure cancer in humans.

As this therapy proved effective and started to save human lives. What was Dr. Burzynski's reward? He was arrested and threatened in court with imprisonment. It seems he had not requested approval from the Food and Drug administration. This can take $4,000.00 and as

98

much as ten years. In the interim, people would die. He was also accused of interstate commerce.

On January 6, 1997, it was clear at the trial that the F.D.A. wanted to jail Dr. Burzynski as a warning to scientists not to use a drug until the F.D.A. approved it.

The irony of this is that Burzysnki had been given interstate permits by the F.D.A. because of pressure from congress– a hung jury.

A trial in May of 1997 resulted in acquittal and thus ended fourteen years of war against Dr. Burzynski for the F.D.A. The government had shown no interest in helping cancer victims. It just wanted to protect its own power.

ABOUT THE AUTHOR

Anne Becker is the pen name of a writer who has traveled extensively. Mrs. Becker did in-depth research in order to write this book. She also does animal welfare work.

Printed in the United States
2869